BLOO
TEARS
& IV'S

BLOOD TEARS & IV'S

*Memoirs of a
Combat Medic
in Operation
Iraqi Freedom*

ELISSA LONSDALE-SMITH

TATE PUBLISHING
AND ENTERPRISES, LLC

Published by Tate Publishing & Enterprises, LLC
127 E. Trade Center Terrace | Mustang, Oklahoma 73064 USA
1.888.361.9473 | www.tatepublishing.com

Tate Publishing is committed to excellence in the publishing industry. The company reflects the philosophy established by the founders, based on Psalm 68:11,
"The Lord gave the word and great was the company of those who published it."

Book design copyright © 2014 by Tate Publishing, LLC. All rights reserved.
Cover design by Jim Villaflores
Interior design by Jimmy Sevilleno

Published in the United States of America

ISBN: 978-1-63367-399-1
Biography & Autobiography / Military
14.08.19

For Michael Yashinski, Craig Ivory, and all the service men and women within every branch who paid the ultimate sacrifice for our country.

CONTENTS

ACKNOWLEDGMENTS

MY FAMILY, WITHOUT your support I wouldn't have made it through. Chuck Dean, for your help and encouragement with this book, and my late brother Fred, always my angel looking over my shoulder.

PREFACE

THE BLOODY AFTERMATH is washed away now, and all that's left is the fog.

Many nights I sit and ponder recent memories of blood and tears shed over the many fallen comrades of an ungodly war we are in. Many times I wonder why we are even here. I remember the dense fog hovering one night as the moon made its descent. I stared intensely into that fog trying to make sense out of this whole thing. Sometimes I still stare into the nothingness and can't see a thing...

A VERY HOT WELCOME

THE DAY I stepped foot into Iraq was the hottest day of my life. Ironically it was the Fourth of July, 2003. I dragged all three of my bags about fifty feet off the rusty old C-130 aircraft, which carried myself and twenty other paratroopers of the 173d Airborne Brigade. Though we were of all different ethnics, backgrounds, jobs, and familiarities, one common thing loomed in the back of our minds—the unknown. I was so afraid of not knowing what to expect. I prayed for God to lead and guide me through this challenging experience. I thought about ten million things all at once, and then the heat interrupted my thoughts.

It felt as though I was standing directly in the exhaust system of the airplane, then I realized it was shut down. We were ordered through a warehouse to a staging area. It felt as though every step I took, it got hotter outside. I later learned that even though it was 9 p.m., the temperature was still at 110 degrees Fahrenheit. My mouth was so dry it felt as though I would swallow my tongue.

I lay on the pavement to get some shut-eye, realizing that sleeping on the concrete floor was a relief to the heat that was blazing outside. Exhausted from the nearly ten hours of travel, I was out like a light within minutes of lying down.

When the call came, I was so overwhelmed by the heat that I was awake even before they started yelling at us to get up.

"You are all going to your units today. Make sure you grab all your baggage and wait outside for your escorts." Selfishly, I just wanted to wash my face and brush my teeth but did what I was told.

Some of the soldiers I had flown in with were brand new to their units. My situation was different. I had been in a school in the States for four months and came out here with the understanding that things were probably going to be a bit strange and uncomfortable at first. Boy, was I right!

When my squad leader arrived to pick me up, I could tell from the look on his face how much my platoon had already been through. They say looks mean everything, and in his case I would say that was a lot. I threw my bags in the back of the Humvee, wiped the sweat off my forehead, and climbed in.

THE SANDPIT

I COULD SEE it a mile away. They called it "the sandpit," and it couldn't have been closer to the truth. Medics in the field are always stationed in strategic places to receive the wounded and care for them; the sandpit was our place. Our aid-station tents were set up in a perimeter-style circle in the middle of a field of sand. There was a picnic table in the center, and they called it "the courtyard." *Funny to have a courtyard with no grass*, I thought.

My squad leader proceeded to give me the grand tour.

"Here we have the pissers, but only for the guys" he nonchalantly pointed out when we got to the latrine facilities. These were simply hollow net poles with plastic bottles cut open and jammed on their ends. The guys used these out in the open, and the poles were dug so the urine would sink three feet into the ground. Then came the wooden port-a-potty. I gasped when I saw all the bugs that had already invaded it. I thought to myself, *I suppose I'll get used to it.* I couldn't have been more right about that.

The squad leader then escorted to me to where my sleep tent was, and I dropped off my gear. I'm always amazed at the camaraderie that exists in an elite unit like the 173d Airborne. We all went the extra mile to look out for one another, and my fellow medics had already set up a cot for me just inside the door flap. It was a small, tight space, but it was *my* space, and I appreciated it so much. Dropping my bags, I continued with my tour.

Being warned of limited water supplies, I grabbed a bottle and tried not to drink it too fast. And then thinking of water, I then asked the question that put a funny look on my squad leader's face.

"What about the shower point?"

He then guided me into this small tin shack that was obviously there before we moved in. I stepped onto a pallet and saw a poncho hanging up with green 550 cord. Behind the magic poncho was the "shower point"—an upside-down orange Coleman's bucket with the spigot cut out. On the ground sat two five-gallon water cans. In order to take a shower, one had to lift this five-gallon water can above one's head and fill the Coleman's bucket. You then wet yourself a little, soap up, and rinse.

I almost cried when I thought of what my buddies had been going through. Something as simple as a good shower could probably restore so much for them. (The infantry troops in the field sometimes went entire weeks without bathing at all.) It made me sad to think of it, and I felt guilty for not going through what they had endured this whole time since being in northern Iraq.

We made our way inside the treatment tent. This was, of course, the most important tent, because it was where all the casualties of war were to be treated. In the heat, however, it is preferred to treat them outside as there is no air conditioning and the tent will get very hot in extreme temperatures. Inside, the treatment area was set up with four litters (the military form of a civilian ambulance stretcher); two on each side. There is a "jumpstart" table in the center of the tent, which contains the defibrillator and intubation equipment. Rumor was that it had only been used once, so far.

The CP, or command post, is of course where the top dogs are. Our platoon leader, Captain Ryan, was always at or near his desk waiting for something to happen—good or bad. He was indeed the mastermind of the operations. The platoon sergeant, SSG Miller, who was in charge of all the enlisted soldiers, was the one to delegate all the decisions made from the command. Though they seemed shocked to see me, I was told they had been expecting me for some time now. Aside from their looks, I took a degree of pride in that comment.

I left the CP and went on to mingle with my fellow medics. I asked questions, got looks, asked questions, got laughs, asked more questions, and was simply told by one medic, "It really sucks here." I knew from the exhausted sunburned look on his face that it was true. *This was not going to be a picnic.*

AWAKEN TO REALITY

FOR THE FIRST two nights in Iraq, I saw no casualties, only sick-call patients during the day—the usual sore throat, minor cuts, scrapes, flu-like symptoms, and mostly diarrhea. Our patient-holding tent held up to twenty patients on cots, and a medic was needed to constantly man it. The water in Iraq was not purified and we were briefed not to drink it. So what did we do? We brushed our teeth in it, and as a result, we found ourselves running to the wooden port-a-potty frequently.

I integrated within my squad but still felt like an outsider because I hadn't been "down-range" (in the war zone) for any length of time, and they had. Our experiences were not on equal footing and it made a difference, so I sat back and observed. I paid attention to every little detail, which proved to be very helpful as time went on.

Sleeping most nights was difficult in the summer because the heat was so unbearable. It soared to 120 during the day and hovered in the 90s at night. The second night I was there, then fiancé, Billy, showed up with a thin Iraqi mattress for my cot and a fan to cool me off at night. He was always looking out for me, no matter where we were.

Billy was in the same brigade but a different unit. He was a team leader in the Ranger's 74th Long-Range Surveillance Detachment. He was a hard worker and very busy with his troops but still made time for me. Bringing me this fan was by far the most morale booster I have seen yet. It would take months for care packages from my family to arrive here. It helped comfort me more than anything. I would lie with that fan turned on me that only seemed to blow hot air in my face, but the thought made me smile.

My dad said he was going to send me a small water bottle fan. Then I could fill it with water and spray it on my face. Maybe that would help me sleep. My sleep deprivation was only just beginning, however.

"Nine line, nine line," I heard some yelling after just dozing off to sleep, and I stirred after realizing where I was. The flap of the tent flew open, and I knew what it all meant. A nine-line medevac request meant we had casualties flying in via medevac helicopter—time to go to work.

Pulling our uniforms on, we hustled to the treatment tent and began setting up saw benches. These were used to throw the medic-ready bags over. We opened up our treatment equipment and waited in a readiness position. Field dressings, Kerlix wrap, Tubex gauze, 4 × 4 pads, thermometers, blood pressure cuffs, stethoscopes, IV bags, needles, syringes, etc.—everything was ready. Someone ordered me to run and grab some five-gallon water cans for the "aftermath." These would be used to wash away the blood after it was all over.

Within fifteen minutes of prepping, we heard the birds (we use the terms 'birds' when referring to military helicopters such as blackhawks) but not see them. It was dark, and the spotlight over our treatment area was so bright that it was impossible to see the night sky anyway. Sergeant Brokenborough, operating the field loading ambulance, was quickly on his way to meet the chopper. Within minutes the casualties were within site, and I didn't know what to expect. I do remember what I was told—*the nine-line information at times would be incorrect.* So we could expect anything—just be ready.

There were two soldiers, both men in their twenties. It was the first of what would be many horrifying sights. They were involved in a shoot out in a town called Fallujah. Both had been shot in the feet with partial amputations. Even though I had been a medic for six years, I had never actually seen anything this bloody, and I almost lost my stomach. I looked around and saw that the other medics were confident and professional in what they were doing, and either the doctor or the senior ranking noncommissioned officer delegated tasks. My squad leader asked me to grab the irrigation solution and start irrigating. No big deal, until the blood started to spurt everywhere.

The fear and anxiety were evident on the soldiers' faces. "You're gonna be all right, don't worry. We'll take care of you and get you outta here," I kept saying to them.

One was telling me not to call his parents because they're in Vegas on vacation. I was thinking, *How selfless this poor kid is, worrying about ruining his parents' vacation.* I wanted to give him a big hug but figured that was just the woman in me.

We irrigated, patched, and reassured the casualties. Then they were on their way to Landstuhl, Germany. This was the major hospital in Europe seeing all the casualties from Iraq, Kuwait, and Afghanistan. In the first three months of the war, Landstuhl had treated more than three hundred casualties.

After the soldiers were gone, the chore of cleaning up the big bloody mess began. The other medics were quick on their toes and knew exactly where everything went. I was so caught up in getting the blood off the pavement it irritated me. As much as I tried to steel myself against what I was doing, I couldn't stand to see the blood that came from these two soldiers' gunshot wounds. It pinched my stomach, and I had to hold my breath to avoid throwing up the contents of my T-rations.

This went beyond my job and what I had trained to do. I had to reach inside and pull up unfamiliar coping ideas, and I had to replace emotions with strength. As I was cleaning up the blood and picking up the soaked bandages and pieces of skin, I prayed to God to give me that strength. I asked him to help me overcome the emotional feelings that I would be having regularly for the next nine months.

DAILY BLOOD

CASUALTIES WERE A routine. It was almost daily by mid-September. This was a bad month. There were rugged enemy Iraqis called guerillas who were "Pro-Saddam" hiding outside our gates, intermingled with the farmers, and just waiting for their opportunity. They would set up roadside bombs called improvised explosive devices (IEDs). They would wait until our infantrymen were out patrolling the streets to start throwing grenades and firing mortar rounds. As of yet, I hadn't experienced any of those things but I knew it was coming. I could feel it.

It all seemed so overwhelming, but I knew I had a job to do and to 'suck it up'. This is a term commonly used in the military to just deal with it.

One day I was cleaning my laundry by hand and a cloud of sand flew into my eyes. I could not see for a minute, and my thoughts raced about those who have lost their eyesight out here. It was a clearly vivid thought. I knew somewhere out there was a soldier who had no sight because of this war. It made me very sad. I put my headphones on and listened to the Beatles; their music helped me through some very depressing situations those first two months.

The blood didn't bother me as much anymore. Now it was more of the faces of the casualties. I could tell how they were feeling and what they were thinking just by looking at them. I would constantly be the one to talk to them. A lot of the time we would get so carried away with treating them that we would forget to keep talking to them. I made that a personal quest to make sure that I had a conversation going with whoever could speak.

Then the war got a little too close. We received a nine-line that turned out to be a friend of mine. His name was Sergeant Danny Pilo. He was on the plane with me when I flew in and was returning to Iraq after his leave home when his little girl was born. I had long talks with him about her, and he was such a proud father.

When he arrived at aid station with a gunshot wound to the foot, he grabbed my hand and said, "Well, at least I get to go home now and see my baby girl." He was smiling and grateful—hole in the foot and all. It was touching.

The realization that I may know someone who comes in for treatment dawned on me, and a certain fear struck me.

Who would be the next? I didn't want to see any more casualties, let alone anyone I knew or was close to. Danny was not afraid, nor would admit he was in any pain. Of course, he was being a man, but he was also being a tough soldier. I told him he would be going home for a little while, and you could see his face getting red. He pulled my sleeve and asked if there was any way he could get back out there with his guys. "Doubtful Danny," I calmly said. He was obviously disappointed.

This bloody routine carried on for a few days in a row and then stopped. We all got rested up knowing it would happen again. I compared it to a "rush" at a supermarket I used to work at. There would be certain days during the week when it would be very slow that you would be bored to tears. Then as the weekend approached, the rush would flood the store. It would be crazy for those few days, and you were so busy you could hardly take a break to eat something. That's what our duty turned into.

The next influx of wounded came in a few days, and it included a few of my buddies from the brigade. They came in by ground evacuation, so I knew it was something that had happened close to our camp. An improvised explosive device (IED) had detonated on a truck full of infantry troops. They did not have any cover and no sandbags on their floorboards, which we were later instructed to do for safety reasons.

When they arrived, I was surprised to see how serious their injuries were. Shrapnel wounds everywhere—it was hard to find them all. The shrapnel looked like scattered splinters all over their faces and necks. The bigger pieces were under their arms probably where the improvised body armor failed to cover. Their legs were covered with small pieces also. The only shrapnel we were real concerned with were the larger pieces in their faces. We had to meticulously remove several pieces of their shrapnel, leaving them scarred for life. Some of the casualties had to stay with us for a week or so to get their dressings changed daily. The brigade chaplain and brigade commanding officers were visiting them. Then they were all awarded the Purple Heart in the patient-holding tent—the first of what would be many awards given to casualties.

CARING FOR THE ENEMY

THE FIRST TIME I saw an Iraqi casualty, I wasn't prepared for how I was going to feel. I knew by the Geneva Convention we had to treat them fairly. I also knew this would bother me if I knew they were firing at or trying to harm one of our own. Three soldiers came in from our 503rd Infantry Battalion. They had gunshot wounds and shrapnel. About ten minutes after they arrived, the wounded enemy Iraqis (who were shooting at our troops) were brought in. They were shot up pretty badly too and screaming in pain. I remember one of the infantry casualties saying he recognized one of the Iraqis from the field when they were firing at them. He wanted to get up and hit him.

The tension was so high we had to move the Iraqis outside to work on them. This was the first "mass cal," or mass casualties situation, that I had seen in-theater. It was very hard to treat the Iraqi men the same as our guys. It was nerve-racking. They would say things like, "You must give me water." Knowing very well all about the Geneva Convention, we *did*, in fact, have to give them food, water, and shelter regardless of what we thought of them or what they had done. You could tell once you got the Iraqi isolated how *few* baths they had taken. The stench was *atrocious at times*, almost unbearable. I would have to cover my face at times just to render follow-up care. We had a small concrete building about one thousand meters away from the main aid station, called the EPW building, set up just for *enemy prisoners of war* and civilian Iraqi casualties. This not only secluded them from our US soldiers but also provided an area to sustain their medical care that wouldn't affect our normal routine. We would treat their serious injuries when they arrived, and then we would send them to the EPW building with a medic and a guard. Usually, the guard is provided the military police or the unit that brought in the soldier.

We had an EPW one day who was very uncooperative. He was fighting and yelling in Arabic, so we brought in the interpreter. Our interpreter Ahmed was very good. He was calm and would let us know word for word what he was saying. We trusted him as one of our own.

The casualty was screaming about his brother. He wanted to go find his brother because he was still "out there" fighting somewhere. He thought it was "unfair" that we had him there. Little did he know, once he was all fixed up, we would ship him over to the detention facility on camp. He would sit there and go through some extensive questioning before they would transport him to the major prison in Baghdad.

A lot of the Iraqi casualties would fight. I think it is only because they aren't used to people taking care of them. They probably also think we're all out to hurt them, which just isn't true. There is a real appeal to treating someone who doesn't exactly like you. It makes you feel like the better man, in a sense.

They can come in and yell, spit, throw things; but all in all, we are doing our job, and they won't do anything to stop us, even if it means restraining them. One EPW had come in, and as my fellow medics were trying to give him pain medicine in his IV, he tried to grab the syringes and stab anyone he could with them. When I heard of this, I was shocked and disgusted all at the same time. How can they not know we are helping them? The Iraqis I felt real sorry for were the innocent civilians caught in the cross-fire. They came in confused, terrified, and sometimes mad. We would explain to them we were going to treat them and they would be released, but a lot of the time they still wanted answers. "Why?" was a common word among the innocent. It was not because we had our own intentions like they thought; it was because we are at war and this is what happens. Regardless of the situation and how difficult it was, we always did the right thing and treated the Iraqis appropriately.

NUNSHAD

HER NAME WAS Nunshad. She was six years old and had been shot in the arm by accident.

There comes a point in your life where you sit back and analyze everything. That day for me was in August. I knew I would eventually deal with injured children, but it was just something that didn't happen very often in our aid station.

I was sitting reading a medical note when three (escorted) Iraqis arrived. One was a man who looked unharmed and was leading them in. The other man had very loose stitches climbing from his chin all the way up to his scalp. The third person was a tiny beautiful girl.

I stared at her for a moment and then realized she was holding her arm in some kind of wrapped bandage. The medics who escorted them in were from a different unit and stated they had been seen at an Iraqi hospital en route here. It is very sad that our tent facility was considered higher quality than their hospital.

I learned that the man with the stitches was her uncle and the other man was her uncle's friend who was driving the car. Apparently they had been driving toward a military checkpoint and decided to turn around to avoid it. The guards at the checkpoint thought this was peculiar so they opened fire on them. One bullet hit the windshield, one skimmed her uncle's head, and he other went right through her poor little arm. It was so sad.

They brought the interpreter in, and he was trying to calm Nunshad down so she can speak. She looked so frightened. Her dress was covered with little pink flowers and splattered with blood, and there was her arm—bandaged and soaked crimson all the way through.

One of our medics tried to tend to her but she backed away. I approached her and asked the interpreter to tell her what I was saying. I asked her if I could look at her arm and that I am not going to hurt her. He then told me what she said: "I only want *her* to help me." I was touched. I looked around and realized that I was the only female in the tent and she must have been uncomfortable with the men.

As I unwrapped her bandage, she stared at me through tear-drenched eyelashes. I could tell she was studying this strange American woman. I was as gentle as I could be. At this point, I had her distracted so the doc could get an IV in her little arm. She would need some good pain medicine for the irrigating of her wound. She was still whimpering and in pain but the medicine's effect soon quieted her. We washed out the hole in her arm and thanked God that the bullet had gone all the way through and missed the bone entirely. I held the sad little girl's hand and comforted her the best I could. We called for further evac at that point.

While we waited for an ambulance, I was touched to see so many of our medics were coming in and offering candy, stuffed animals that someone had sent from home, and water and food. It was unbelievable how many people cared so deeply because it was a child. I understood that this was a big accident and my outlook on the whole thing was different than when we saw EPWs (enemy prisoners of war). I truly felt her pain and confusion.

That incident changed me. It was the deepest feeling I had felt in a long time. She uncovered something in me—my need to help the children. I wanted to get out there and go on these medical-capability missions that were about two a month. The doctors would take a couple of medics out and go to the clinics and hospitals to help give medical aid to those in need. That was my next goal. I had to do it for myself.

A HOSPITAL FROM HELL

NOT MANY DAYS later, I was selected for a medical-capability (or med caps) mission to the local Kirkuk General Hospital. I made sure my medical bag was fully stocked and my camera was in my pocket. I was feeling excited but nervous and wasn't sure what to expect. I had heard some horrible things about their own medical care.

We drove by Humvee the twenty-minute drive to the hospital area. As we came to a traffic circle, I saw a sight that only a war and poverty could produce. The hospital was completely torn apart. The walls looked like they were falling apart from the outside, and the street leading into the hospital was flooded with pedestrians, many of whom looked as though they needed medical care. In addition to this, there were others simply loitering, which, in a combat arena such as Iraq, is never good.

As we drove along, it felt like we were in a parade. Children ran loose in the streets and hooted and hollered when they saw us driving by in the Humvees. They would run alongside us and yell. Of course, I had no idea what they were saying, but they seemed excited to see us. *Maybe it's because we are so different,* I thought.

As for the scenery, I found nothing special to look at in this country—just a lot of dirt, trash, and torn-apart shacks for homes—but I was hoping my impression would some-day change.

As we walked up to the entrance of the hospital, an Iraqi doctor greeted us. Dr. Abib-Rashr seemed very nice and willing to show us around. I noticed right away his over-coat, which probably once used to be white, was a stained, dirty off-color now. His teeth were streaked with stains of black tar, and his eyes were dry and hollow rounds. I thought, *Man it's pretty bad when the doctor is unhealthy.*

The hospital reeked of sweat. It smelled like a gym after a basketball game. I smiled and hoped that my displeasure for the stench would go unnoticed. The first floor was filled with people waiting to be seen. I hardly saw any rooms or doctors that weren't occupied. The elevator was broken, so we took the stairs. After letting them know that I wanted to see the children, they took me to the Pediatrics on the fourth floor.

As we walked in, I almost fell over at what I saw. Right in front of the premature babies' room was a female doctor, smoking a cigarette, leaning over an open incubator! In the next room, we came to a woman holding her infant. The baby was barely big enough to fit in the palm of your hand. She was just rocking her and looked up at me with such happiness. I thought, *If this woman only knew the medical care her baby was missing.*

The doctor explained (in English) that woman's infant was a premature baby and had been born two days earlier at only seven months of gestational pregnancy. She seemed oblivious to how dangerous that was. He also explained how common this was in Iraq. As we made our way to the children's ward, I became more and more troubled by what I was seeing.

At the children's ward, none of the beds had sheets on them. None of the IV (intravenous infusion) poles had IV bags on them, and the shelves looked bare. As expected, the children were very malnourished. One in particular caught my eye. He was a small boy lying so still I thought he was dead. His head was swollen to the size of a watermelon. I asked the doctor what was wrong with him, and he explained that the boy had a subdural hematoma. He went on to explain that the child would probably die because they didn't have the resources to take care of it.

Chills went up my spine partly because the doctor was so nonchalant about it.

The next bed we came to held a tiny girl. She was three, according to the doctor, but looked much younger. She was just so small. I figured her to be a year old at best.

Doctor Abib said she needed a bone-marrow transplant and that they couldn't do that in Iraq. He said they were trying to find the funds to transfer her to Afghanistan because it is possible there.

"How good are the chances?" asked one of our doctors.

"Very slim," replied Doctor Abib sadly.

I realized how much we take for granted. We complain about waiting in lines to get the luxuries that are afforded to us, or that we may be charged more than we bargained for. Most Americans never realize how good we have it. We are alive, healthy, and well taken care of. As I stood in that hospital, my heart became more and more troubled, and I felt different about the life we have in America.

FULLY LOCKED AND LOADED

WHEN WE WERE outside of the camp, we were always locked and loaded. Though I never had to pull the trigger, there were times when I thought I would.

There is nothing like the feeling you get in the back of the truck with ten to twenty other soldiers, all who have loaded weapons. While you are all pointed outward, you have not only a sense of security but also a fear something terrible could go wrong.

My point was proven one day when a private was rushed in with a terrible wound. He had just come back from a mission and was clearing his 50-caliber rifle before entering the camp. He reported that he had misfed a round and when he went to clear it, another one pushed it out and into his foot. He had a hole in his foot probably about six inches wide, nearly the entire width of his foot.

I knew that this had to be a lesson for all to learn, and I gathered as many people as I could so they could see the effects of reckless clearing. The soldier obviously was pointing the weapon at his foot instead of out and away like we were all taught.

The improvised explosive devices on the sides of the roads became such a big issue that we were told if an Iraqi comes up to your truck while you're stopped, you can point your weapon at him and tell him to leave. If he is persistent, you must fire before he gets a chance to slide a bomb under your truck. That was a scary thought to me because it seemed like they were all so curious and wanting to come up to you. I feared having to take that action on innocent human beings.

Then there were the kids. They would stand on the side of the road and throw apples and oranges in the back of our trucks. We were told they were doing this for "grenade" practice. Aiming and testing to see at which angle and what technique would be needed to make sure that the grenades went into the back of moving Army vehicles. It hurt inside when I thought about innocent children who are misdirected in their behavior by grown-ups who use them for their own agendas.

For every mission I went on, I saw at least twenty-five Iraqis who actually looked suspicious of something. Maybe it was the way they looked at us, or just their body language. I didn't feel comfortable looking directly at them unless they were small children. The children always seemed so excited to see us. It was as if we were movie stars straight out of Hollywood. I couldn't imagine how these young kids could be so influenced to hurt Americans. I didn't understand it for a long time, and then one day it became clear to me.

I was on a medical-capability mission to a clinic. We were walking through the streets of a small town giving medical aid while making our way to the clinic. These children were all over us and following us everywhere. They came up to me and pointed at things on my uniform, such as a flashlight or my bandage scissors, and ask what they are for. One kid had the audacity to actually grab my sunglasses right off my body armor, and subconsciously I began to put on a different kind of armor—distrust.

The kids had a lot of energy. Many were yelling out a chant as we walked around town. Curious as to what they were saying, I asked our interpreter what it all meant.

He explained that it translated to, "Saddam will reign again." I could not believe my ears and thought of the irony. These kids either really didn't understand what they were saying, or perhaps I was just so naive that I didn't realize how smart they really were.

Needless to say, it would be most difficult to ever shoot a child. I am not wired that way. If ever it came to a heated moment in wartime and I had to pull the trigger that took a young life, I could probably never forgive myself. No matter how brainwashed that child may be, I still would find it hard to get over. It is inconceivable to me that such a young soul could be so desensitized by the ravages of war. It saddened my heart even more to think of how their lives are forever changed by the devastation around them.

IVORY

THERE WERE FIVE soldiers in my squad, and I want to take a moment to mention them. We all worked very well as a team. I was the team leader who actually spent more time with them than their actual squad leader. We bonded through a lot of hands-on training and spent some of our down time together. During the summer, the pool at camp was our favorite hangout. We also enjoyed cookouts occasionally on the hot summer nights, and those of us who smoked cigarettes would hang out at the picnic table.

One of these soldiers was Specialist Craig Ivory. When I first got to Iraq, he slept in the cot next to mine. He was the first one I would wake every morning by kicking his bunk. Not a very deep sleeper, he would jump out of bed at the first kick of my boot on his cot leg. Ivory was a caring and motivated individual. He had a lot of drive and made things happen. He was up for missions off-camp as well as on. He had a unique personality. You could hear his obnoxious laugh a mile away.

In mid-August, I had radio watch duty (this is called RTO—radio transmission operator), and Ivory and the other guys were running the treatment tent. They had been pulling sick call for a few hours. The day seemed normal with nothing chaotic so far.

Suddenly, I heard a thud from the tent next door. I ran to the tent and saw Ivory laid out on the floor. Previously I learned, he had started shaking and running in circles looking for something. He was out of his head and could not tell anyone what it was looking for. As soon as I entered the tent, I saw him convulsing. I knew we had to get him out of there, and fast.

I got on the radio and informed the Air Force we were evacuating a patient over to their facilities. I explained that he had possible seizures and unconsciousness. Ivory was put in the back of our field loading ambulance (FLA) and taken over to their emergency ward. The Air Force was the next level of care because they had better high-tech equipment. From there, Specialist Ivory was taken to Landstuhl Hospital in Germany.

I had grown close to him, and this incident was especially upsetting for me. He and I would sometimes sit and talk about his family. He so looked forward to seeing his family again. Ivory was passionate about his bull-riding and cowboy ways. He loved country music and dreamed of buying a jeep with gigantic tires when we got home. He also told me of a girlfriend he had met at the Air Force medical facility. I am amazed how death can bring back so many tender thoughts of the person that has gone on.

Our brigade surgeon, Major Nixon, would update us every night on Ivory's condition, and I held my breath at each session. Ivory ended up in a coma shortly after arriving in Germany. They said he had a blood clot that had traveled from his heart to his brain stem and then lodged itself. It was difficult to believe this was actually happening. Here was a twenty-six-year-old kid, only one year older than me, and he was so close to death this way.

The platoon remained very quiet and reserved for the next few days. Everyone looked sad, and the hollowed eyes told me that they all had that "thousand-mile stare" over the entire incident.

After five intense days of being in a coma, Ivory was taken off the life-support machine. Specialist Craig Steven Ivory was gone. There was nothing we could have done to save him, and that's what tore me apart the most. I still wonder if perhaps we could have caught it earlier or somehow known this was going to happen. I saw no signs, but then again, I wasn't exactly looking for any either. It was just one big surprise. No one was quite sure exactly what could have caused this to happen to him, and this only added to the mystery and bad feelings—we just needed to get some closure.

I did know he was adopted. No one, including him, knew the medical history of his biological parents. They could have had a history of strokes or heart conditions, but there was no way to tell.

I lived in disbelief for the next few days. Several times in the nights to follow, I woke up and looked for him in the cot next to me. It was so weird he wasn't there. He had this obnoxious laugh that I could never ever forget. It used to annoy me, and now I truly missed it. I remembered things he said just the day before. I would replay those things in my mind and almost hear him saying them.

The memorial service had to be that Friday of the week he died. My platoon sergeant asked me if I wanted a role in the service. I selected to write the invocation. I sat down, and it just flowed onto the paper. I went outside and saw seven of my fellow medics practicing the twenty-one-gun salute. I knew they had each volunteered, and it brought tears to my eyes.

When the memorial service came, I was far from being emotionally ready. I had to march up there and open up the service in front of nearly 150 soldiers from the brigade, other units, and the Air Force. As I started speaking, I could feel my palms become clammy and the sweat running down my face. I knew I was not going to be able to do this without tearing up. People were staring so sadly at me and it filled the room as I began:

> Good morning. We are here today to honor Specialist Craig Ivory. Before I begin, I would like to say a few words about him. He was one of the soldiers in my squad, the Airborne Treatment team Alpha. I was his team leader. He was bright and full of energy.
>
> Specialist Ivory was a hard-working and dedicated soldier. He was not afraid to sweat. He took initiative and took pride in all he did. He was in charge of the five-ton truck for our squad. He took great pride in fixing it up. If something needed to be done, he'd stay at the motor pool half the night and come back covered in grease and oil, but the mission would be complete.
>
> Specialist Ivory was an outstanding medic. He would show concern and care toward patients no matter how small or big their problem might be. He would always volunteer to be the on-call medic at night and to go out on dangerous missions. He wanted to see the action. He wanted to be a part of everything.
>
> He was a great person who cared sincerely about those around him, even those he did not know. He had made a friend in the Air Force. Her name is Misty. I would like her to know if she is here today that he talked very highly of her. If you asked any-

one about Specialist Ivory, they would all say the same thing: He had a heart of gold.

He lived life. He had hopes and dreams. He showed me pictures of the Jeep Wrangler he wanted to buy when he got back to Texas, with monster-size tires. He listened to country music, was a big fan of Hank Williams, Jr.; he even brought his cowboy boots out here with him. He loved bull riding, line dancing, and *Buffy the Vampire Slayer*. His hobbies include wrestling and working out.

Specialist Craig Ivory was a great person, a proud soldier, and will always remain in our hearts and minds. He will never be forgotten.

Please rise for the invocation:

I would like to read a scripture from the Old Testament:

> There is a time for everything and a season for every activity under heaven. A time to be born and a time to die, a time to plant and a time to uproot, a time to kill and a time to heal, a time to tear down and a time to build, a time to weep and a time to laugh, a time to mourn and a time to dance, a time to scatter stones and a time to gather them, a time to embrace and a time to refrain, a time to search and a time to give up, a time to keep and a time to throw away, a time to tear and a time to mend, a time to be silent and

a time to speak, a time to love and a
time to hate, a time for war and a time
for peace.

Ecclesiastes 3:1–8

Let us pray:

Dear Lord,

May you provide comfort and safety to Craig Ivory
in his time of departure. Lord, we ask of you to relieve
him of all troubles and stresses so he can rest peace-
fully. May you rest his soul and ensure he knows just
how truly he is missed. Lord, shed your blessings
on his family. Give them the strength and guidance
that they need through these difficult times. Lord,
bring a sense of understanding to his family and all
who knew him. We trust in your judgment, Lord, as
we will lean on each other for support. Let us learn
to rejoice once we have mourned, for he is in a better place, in your hands. Lord, we ask of these things
in your heavenly name, amen.

BIOGRAPHY OF CRAIG STEVEN IVORY

(Courtesy of Patrick Ivory)

Craig Ivory was born on January 24, 1977, in
Charleston, SC. He was the adopted son of Mr.
Patrick Ivory and Mrs. Mary Kay Ivory. He lived

with his father and step-mother, Teresa Ivory, from the age of ten until he joined the Army in January 1997. Craig attended various schools die to his father being a career naval officer.

He graduated from the State College Area High School in States College, PA. He lettered in track, football, and also played the clarinet and bass clarinets in the symphonic band He also enjoyed wrestling and took up bull riding while I he was stationed in Texas.

SPC Ivory's original Army job title was a light-wheeled vehicle mechanic. He also attended jump school at Fort Benning, Ga. He served a year-long tour in Korea and also at Fort Campbell, KY. He remained at Fort Campbell until he re-enlisted to become a medic. After completing advanced individual training (Combat Medic School), he was stationed at Fort Bliss, TX. Although he loved Texas, he wanted to be in an airborne unit so he again re-enlisted for the 173rd Airborne Brigade, in Vicenza, Italy. He was assigned to the 501st. Forward Support Company Medical Platoon in August 2002. In March 203, Craig was sent with the brigade to Kirkuk, Iraq, in support of Operation Iraqi Freedom. In August 2003, he suffered a stroke and was transferred from Iraq, to Kuwait and then to Landstuhl Army Medical Center in Germany.

He was then transferred to Homburg University Hospital where every effort was made to save him. Due to the severity of the brain injury, he was declared brain dead and was removed from life-support in August 17, 2003. His father and brother, Brandon, were at his side.

SPC Ivory's awards include: The Bronze Star, Army Commendation Medal, Army Achievement Medal, National Defense Service Medal, Parachutist badge, Combat Medical badge, and a marksmanship badge. He was honored by his fellow soldiers after his death when the aid station he worked in was renamed the Ivory Combat Clinic. SPC Ivory was buried with full military honors at Fort Indiantown Gap National Cemetery in Annville, Pennsylvania.

He is survived by his parents, step-mother, brothers Brandon and Sean and sister Amanda. His family loved him very much and is extremely proud of his service to his country. He is sorely missed and thought of often. His father has established a scholarship in his name, specifically for medics and corpsman who are attending a physician assistant program. Craig's father is a physician assistant and one day, Craig had hoped to follow in his footsteps. Additionally, a memorial bench has been placed at his high school alma mater by his family. Inscribed is the bench is, "What we do in life…echoes through eternity. This was one of Craig's favorite quotes ad was written to his family in letters and e-mails home. He has made his mark on this world!

(Courtesy of the Ivory family)

MORALE MOVE

THE PLATOON HAD experienced a tremendous loss. When one of our own goes down, it involved a different set of dynamics of grief and healing. We needed a change.

Change actually came at the perfect time. The platoon leader ordered the relocation of our entire aid station. He arranged for us to be set up closer to the air evacuation unit. He also made sure that were on solid ground with the treatment and command post tents under a permanent concrete bunker.

He was completely right. We did need to move out of the sandpit. Though it gave us a lot more work to do to make this happen, we also realized how good this would be for our morale. With a certain joy and new determination began a vigorous move that took our unit onto the pavement about five hundred meters to our rear. Two days later, we were completely moved, and our morale went out the roof. We all got a fresh start, so to speak.

The tents we moved into were provided by the Air Force, so they were, of course, a lot nicer and better insulated. We were supposed to be getting air-conditioning units soon, so that was a great factor. And for me, I had a new soldier who was now sleeping in the cot next to me. Along with the new location, I knew it would make it easier not to think about Ivory all the time.

The "new" treatment and CP tents were set under a very large concrete bunker to make our patients and us safer from mortar rounds and rocket-propelled grenades. We used to have to do bunker drills underground in the dirt, but now our bunker drills consisted of running into the patient hold on the backside of the treatment tent. There was no more dirt, and the bugs wouldn't be near as bad on the pavement as they were in the sandpit.

Perhaps the best part of the entire move is that we were now right next to the 54th Air Evacuation Team. This asset would make it a lot easier when it came to pushing casualties out to other facilities. Things were looking better all the time.

We were all discussing the good points of the move, not concerned at all with how much work we had just done. I began noticing major mood changes from the other soldiers. The anger and frustration was not as frequent as before. For the first time in a while, I felt a strong bond between the medics and knew we were all leaning on each other for moral support.

After the big move, things seemed to be a lot more organized and cleaner than before. During the month of September, we received bunk beds, followed by air-conditioning units. It just kept getting better and better. But we all knew that this was bound to change and probably meant that something very bad was about to happen.

THE FIRST BODY BAG

THEY SAY THE first dead body will stick with you always. I know now that this is very true.

As I made notes in my journal. I wrote, "I woke this day to feel somewhat refreshed. I knew my peace with Ivory had been made and that he was in heaven smiling down on us. I could feel his presence in the wind. I felt a higher morale level due to the move." This was a brand new day for me in Iraq.

We saw patients during the day and prepared for the worst that night, as always. When the worst came, however, I was not prepared to deal with it.

That first body bag made an indelible mark on my soul. Specialist Mark Kent came to us by air. He was rushed in from yet another IED attack on the Humvee he was riding in. When we took him out of the helicopter, he was already in the final stages of shock. His heartbeat was well over two hundred beats per minute. This was going to be very hard to reverse.

I was told to remove his helmet. He had a large hole in the front of his helmet where a piece of the Kevlar was completely blown out. It was covered in blood and mud. I went to place the helmet on the ground and noticed something that will stay with me forever—a picture of his wife buried deep inside. I looked at it only for a split second but will never forget her face. She was beautiful and smiling. I couldn't help but think, *I'll bet that made him smile every day.*

We tried everything on Mark. We shocked his heart several times; we intubated him and started pushing air into his lungs through a bag-valve mask. Forty-five minutes later, he was pronounced dead by one of our doctors.

Unfortunately, we had to examine him and annotate his injuries and fatal wounds. I noted that one of his fatal wounds was a large piece of shrapnel that the blast had projected into his forehead. He had more fatal wounds in the thigh, stomach, neck, and chest.

I was an emotional wreck but forced myself not to show it. After the note-taking we covered his body with a green Army-issued wool blanket. We made sure his eyes were closed and hands folded together on his stomach. By this time, his entire chain of command was surrounding us and most of his buddies were there. We had quite an audience and quite a disappointment. Although we knew there wasn't much we could have done, it was a horrible and tragic loss.

When someone dies, Mortuary Affairs is notified to take care of the after-death matters. For some reason, it was taking a while for them to respond, so I was selected to stand guard on the body. Four of us grabbed a black body bag and moved Specialist Kent from the blanket into the bag. We zipped it up, securing the handles, and then moved him to the backside of the aid station; out of view from any bystanders.

Once we got him to the rear of the tent, we placed him in front of a berm where the wind would not hit him so much. I sat on a sandbag to watch over him until Mortuary Affairs arrived. Three hours went by and I was still sitting there when one of my fellow medics came over and started talking to me. I broke down, and I cried and cried.

I had never seen a dead body before that was not in a funeral wake coffin. You could smell and feel the death in the air. It was like nothing I had ever felt. It was so surreal that I had thoughts that perhaps this was all a dream and I was about to wake up. What I didn't realize was this was just the beginning of what would become a reoccurring dream.

I sat and stared at the black shiny body bag under the light of the moon. It was suddenly so quiet outside, and I felt as if we could have done more to save him. This kid was twenty-three years old. I just could not believe it.

All of a sudden, I saw his body rise up.

"Oh God! He isn't dead, he isn't dead!" I shouted.

Specialist Charlie Quiroz, sitting next to me, shook my shoulder and asked if I was all right. I was hallucinating. I realized it was not real. I saw him move and sit up, and it took Quiroz a long time to convince me I was seeing things.

Finally, Mortuary Affairs showed up. *Just in time to save my sanity*, I thought.

I will never forget that day, or the look on Mark's face, or the picture of his wife in his helmet. I will never understand why it had to happen to him, or anybody for that matter. Why is death so abrupt and sudden? Why do young people get killed? Why do good people die? These questions may remain a mystery in my mind for a long time.

BIRTHDAY WITH A BANG

AT 2100 (9:00 P.M.) HOURS, October 16, 2003, I was called to the squad tent and given a mission for the next day—which happened to be my twenty-fifth birthday.

"You are to convoy down to Tikrit with the 112th Infantry, 4th Infantry Division. Your mission is to go to the Combat Support Hospital and pick up x-ray film. Easy enough?"

I went back to my tent and started checking my medical bag to make sure it was stocked. I was nervous and had a funny feeling about the convoy to Tikrit on my birthday. Tikrit had a bad reputation for car bombings and IEDs. That night, I prayed, "Please, God, keep us all safe on this trip. Let me be ready and capable if anything should happen."

There were three other soldiers from my company going on this convoy—two males and a female. I was a friend to all of them. They were riding in a five-ton truck; two in the front, and the female was on top operating the machine gun for tightened security in the rear. We picked up class-1 rations to ensure that we had food supplies, and then I climbed in the back of their truck to be near my guys. I faced my locked and loaded rifle out for the two-hour journey to Tikrit.

It never occurred to me that the medic should never ride in the rear of the convoy. Statistically, it was the vehicle with the greatest chance of being bombed or attacked, and if anything happened, I needed to be there ready to take care of casualties—not being one myself! I felt a little stupid and prayed that nothing bad would happen.

We made it to Tikrit in record time. On the way down, we saw suspicious things on the side of the road but nothing too alarming. When I saw a pile of rocks, I figured it was just a "pile of rocks." Once we were there, I completed my mission to the Combat Support Hospital and picked up the x-ray film.

After eating a decent meal for a change in their chow hall, we prepared to reembark on the journey back to Kirkuk. It was about 1600 (4:00 p.m.) hours.

As we were waiting to collect the rest of our convoy, which had separate missions, I had a conversation with the convoy commander, and he agreed I should ride in the first vehicle on the way back.

"Medics should never be in the rear," he said.

As much as I hated to leave my guys, I climbed into the back of *his* Humvee and faced out to pull security. It was a very bright day out, and I knew it was going to be a very hot, long trip home.

It ended up being "hot" in other ways too. We had only driven about an hour when an explosion behind us rang in my ears.

"What the hell was that?" the radio crackled.

"We've been hit! We've been hit! Rear vehicle!"

I could see the smoke and debris flying through the air. I wasn't sure what had happened, but I knew it was not good. Fear and adrenaline rushed through my body.

The captain pulled a fast U-turn and sped back to the explosion.

He looked at me and said, "Okay, Doc, do your thing."

I grabbed my weapon and my aid bag and jumped out of the truck. Running toward the accident seemed like slow motion. On my left, I saw the truck tumbling through the field. I saw the fire, the smoke, and pieces of the truck all over the road. I kept running. I saw infantrymen quickly forming a perimeter. Then I heard the gunshots ringing in my ear. I wasn't sure if we were being attacked, but I knew I had a job to do.

As I ran closer, I saw the bodies. They were spread about twenty feet apart from each other and about a hundred feet from the truck that blazed with fire. All had been thrown from the five-ton truck. They all had to have been knocked unconscious from the impact.

Specialist Rivera was the first person I came to. She was awake but disoriented, and when she saw me, she grabbed my hand and started asking what had happened.

"Calm down, Riv, I'm gonna take care of you."

She was very concerned about where her truck was. Then she mentioned she couldn't see anything without her glasses. I told her not to worry, we would find them later. Right now, I was concentrating on her wounds, especially the shrapnel lodged in her forehead. It had missed her helmet by maybe a quarter of an inch. I grabbed some Kerlix wrap and bandaged her head, and then I did a quick sweep of the rest of her body.

She had another piece of shrapnel lodged behind one of her ankles. It was bleeding profusely, and I applied a pressure dressing followed by a bandage. When I touched her arm and leg, she screamed out in pain. They were so swollen I couldn't tell if they had fractures, so to be safe I proceeded to splint them. I made sure that she stayed as calm as possible and kept talking to me. When I left her, I reassured her that I would be back.

The second casualty I came to was Sergeant Luis. He seemed more alert but obviously in shock. He tried to get up and kept telling me he wanted to check on Rivera. I told him to stay put so I could check him out.

As I conducted the quick assessment I put my bandage scissors to good use. He had no major injuries above his legs. I then came to his thigh, and he squealed out in pain. He had a large piece of shrapnel protruding from his right thigh. The impaled object needed to be secured. I pulled out some gauze and wrapped it first around the shrapnel and taped it in place, and then bandaged the leg to stop the bleeding. I encouraged him to keep talking to Rivera.

Specialist Tucker was the last casualty. He was lying next to the road and was looking around for the truck, and I asked him where he was hurt. He indicated that it was his back. I told him not to move and placed a cervical collar around his neck and then did a rapid trauma assessment and found no further severe injuries.

It was at this point I yelled for someone to call in a nine-line medevac request. I shouted out the injuries: "Possible spinal injury, impaled shrapnel, right thigh, head wound associated with shrapnel, impaled shrapnel wound to the Achilles tendon, possible fractures of the wrist, arm, and leg." Within five minutes, the helicopters were in the air.

I ran back to check on Rivera. She was very confused and kept asking me where her glasses were. I grabbed a private who was standing around and told him to look through the debris for her glasses. Surprisingly she remembered she had a spare pair in her rucksack. That was a relief. It told me her head injury was not that severe.

She was gripping onto me so tight it made me feel a sense of relief. This also told me how strong she still was. She kept asking me if everyone else was all right. "You're all going to make it outta here. Hang in there, Riv." By now the birds had landed.

The flight medics ran up with spine boards. Specialist Tucker was the first to be strapped down due to his possible spinal injury. He was a good sport and stayed still the whole time.

Next was Rivera. She was crying now but was grateful she could see everything. As they took her away, she grabbed my hand and said, "Thank you, Sergeant Lonsdale."

Then Sergeant Luis was placed on a litter and carried off. He still acted like he wanted to help everybody else, careless about his impaled thigh.

With overwhelming emotion and adrenaline, I stood there and watched the birds lift off. It was amazing. I knew those were my buddies and my comrades up there and that they were going to be okay. The feeling of knowing I accomplished my job under these circumstances was incredible.

I picked up the mess I had left and climbed back into the Humvee to head home. We still had a good thirty minutes' driving time to Kirkuk. I was terrified. I kept hearing that bang and seeing that smoke. I was so afraid that it might happen again before we got back.

Luckily, we made it back safely. I was dropped off at the aid station just in time to see my casualties being loaded up to go to Landstuhl Hospital. Gently touching Rivera's arm, I told her to hang in there, and knowing that her fiancé had been contacted and was allowed to go with her was very good because she was an emotional wreck.

Some of the truck drivers came around about that time.

"What happened to the truck?" Specialist Tucker asked.

It amazed me that these truck drivers got blown out of their truck and that's all they were concerned about. I told him it was a wreck but not to worry because he had survived.

Sergeant Luis grabbed my hand and said, "I owe you."

"Hey, Lu, you don't owe me anything. It's my job," I said. And then he was gone.

I sat down and took half of my gear off. I could only sit there for an hour or so, because I was restless. I was in some heavy thought and a mild state of shock over what had just happened. People wanted to talk to me and ask questions, but I just was not ready for that. I still could not believe what had just happened.

A few hours and half a pack of cigarettes later, I was informed that the five-ton truck they were in had been towed back to camp. It was now sitting over at the maintenance bay, and immediately I got up and ran over there to see its condition.

The section that was completely blown out was in the rear of the truck at the exact location where I was sitting on the way down there. *Amazing*, I thought. The entire bench where I sat was gone. The passenger side door was blown out and the rest of that side was charred. The tires bent inward and the .50-caliber machine gun that Rivera was manning was melted to itself.

I couldn't believe where the majority of the damage was. In that very instant, I thanked God for sparing my life. I knew if I had sat in the same location that I had on the way down there, I would probably be dead, and those three casualties wouldn't have had a medic to care for them. *Medics never ride in the rear of a convoy.*

I thanked God for giving me the strength to treat them under the smoke and gunfire. I thanked him for sparing my life on my twenty-fifth birthday. I had called my parents a week later and told them what had happened. It was an amazing story I got in return. It turns out my grandmother had called my step-mom the night before my birthday. She told her she had a bad feeling about me and my birthday. (No one had any idea of the mission I was going on, as we were told not to share information like that over the phone.) So she said a prayer that night to keep me safe on my birthday. I was so grateful she had said that prayer.

The Lord does work in mysterious ways, I thought.

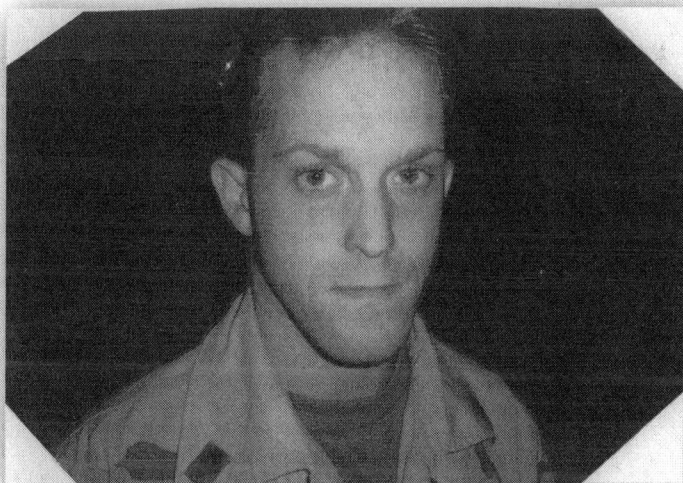

Specialist Craig S. Ivory

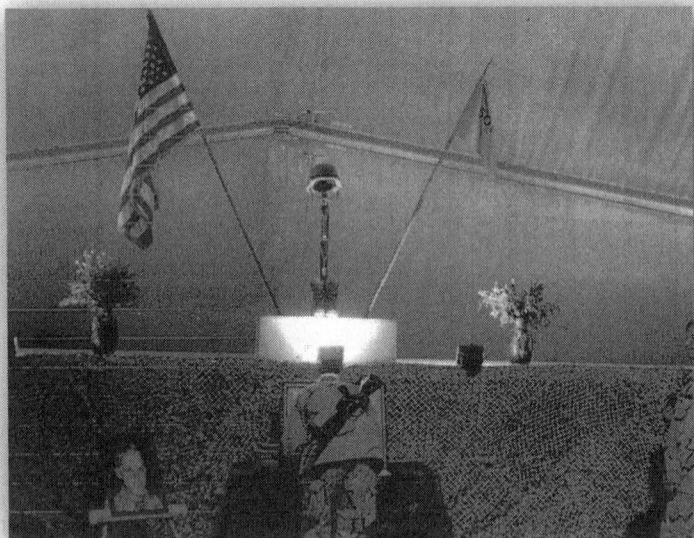

This is the memorial service for Specialist Craig Ivory.

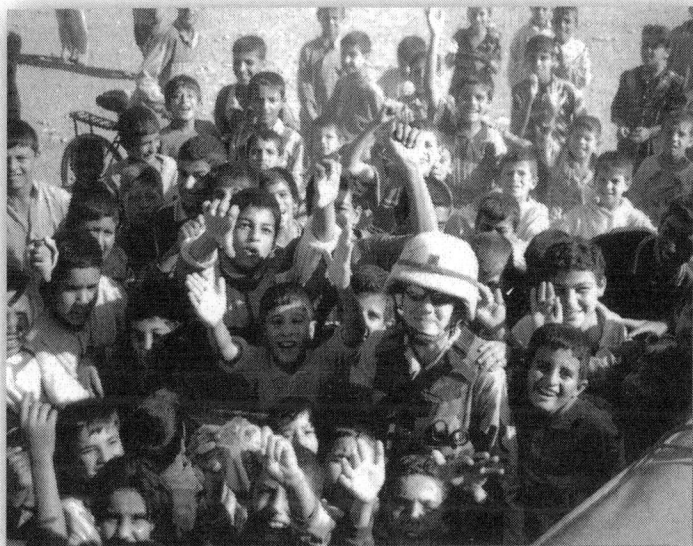

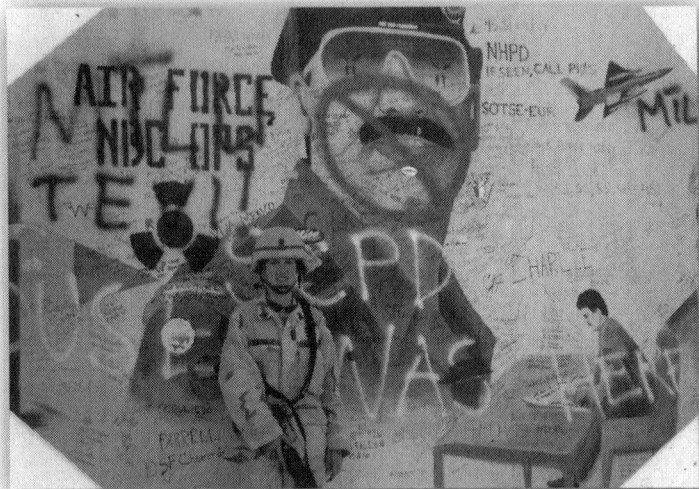

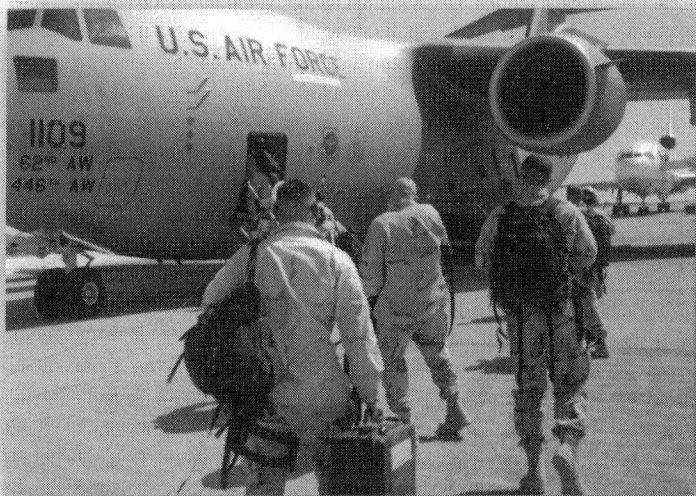

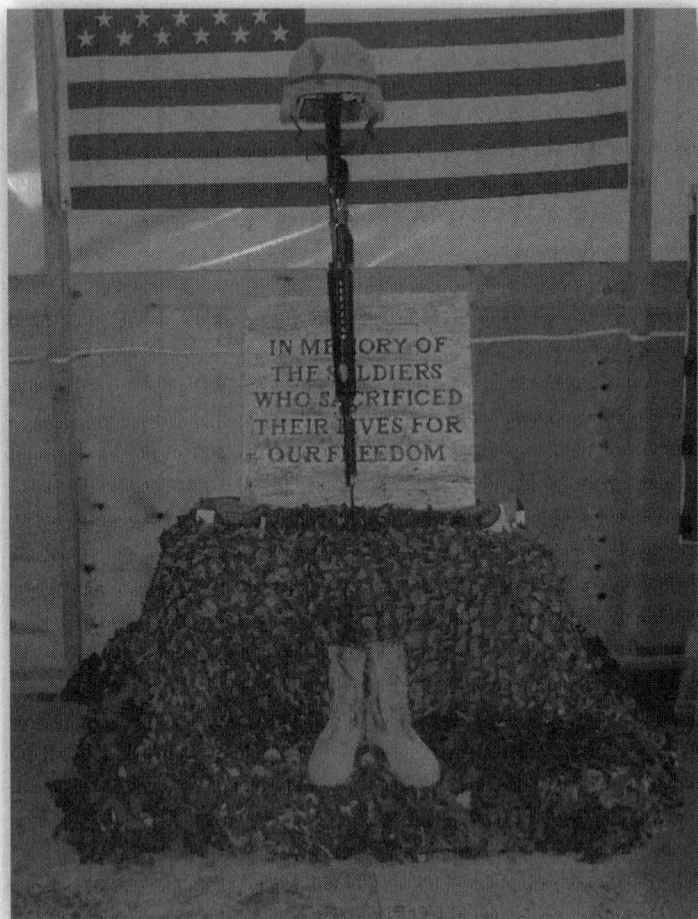

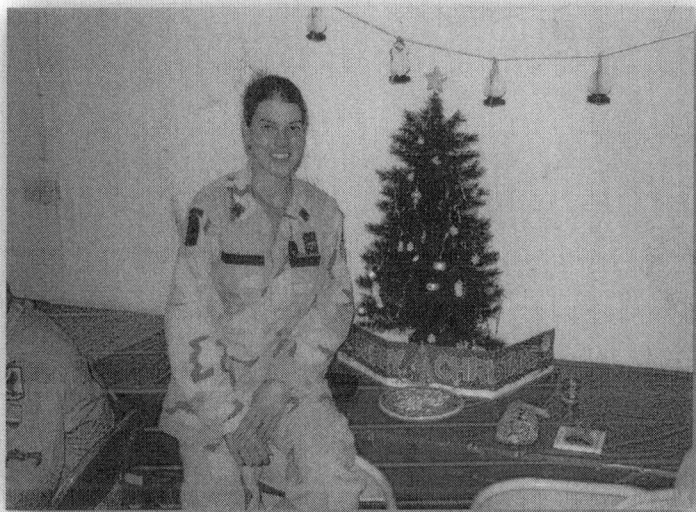

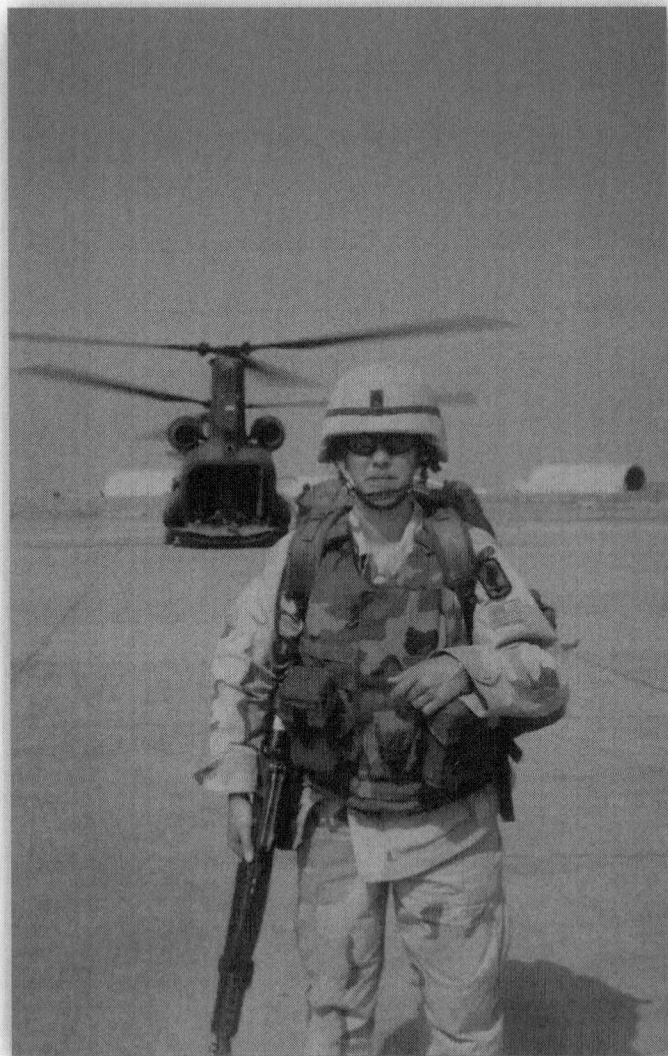

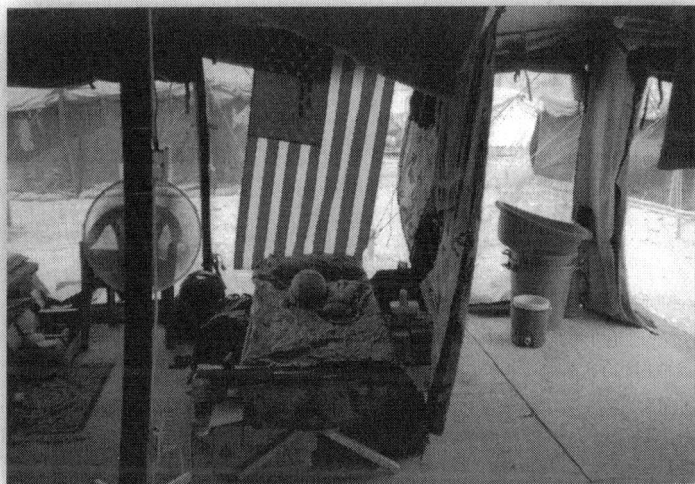

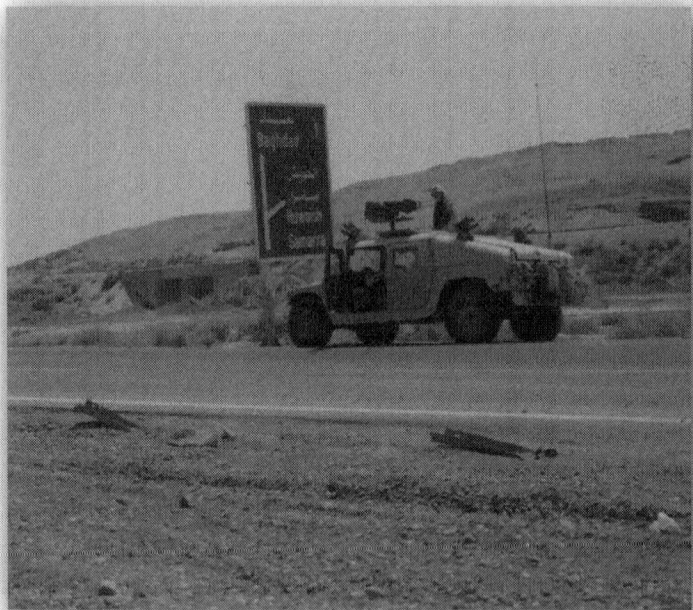

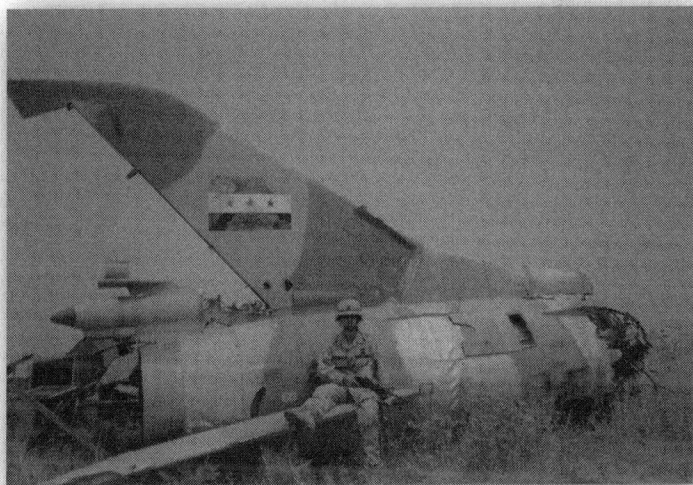

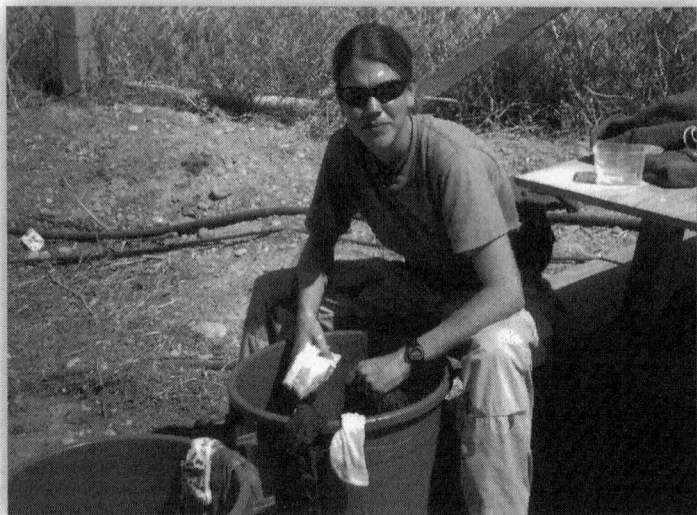

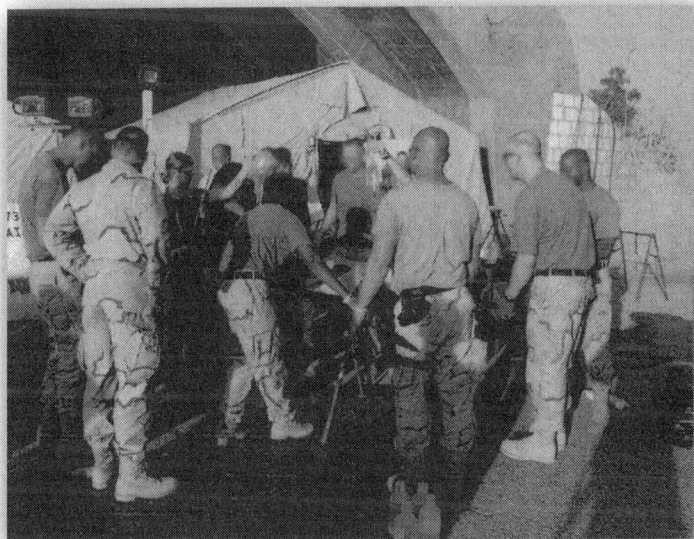

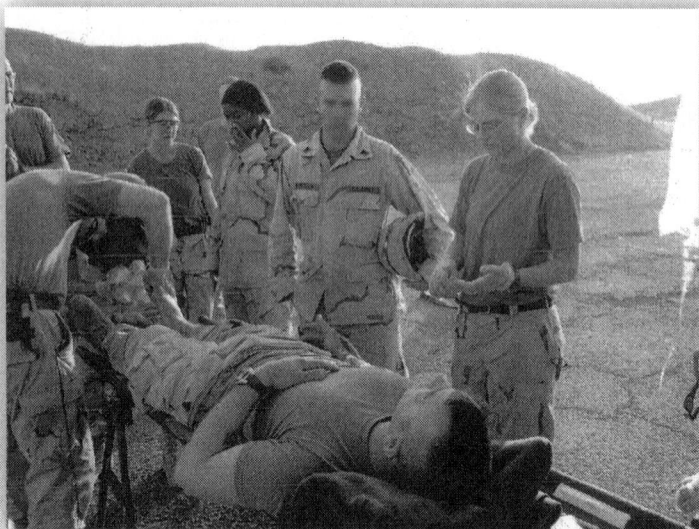

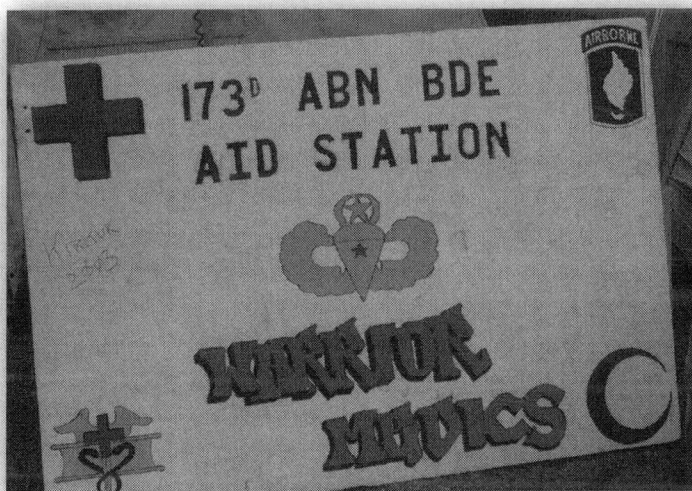

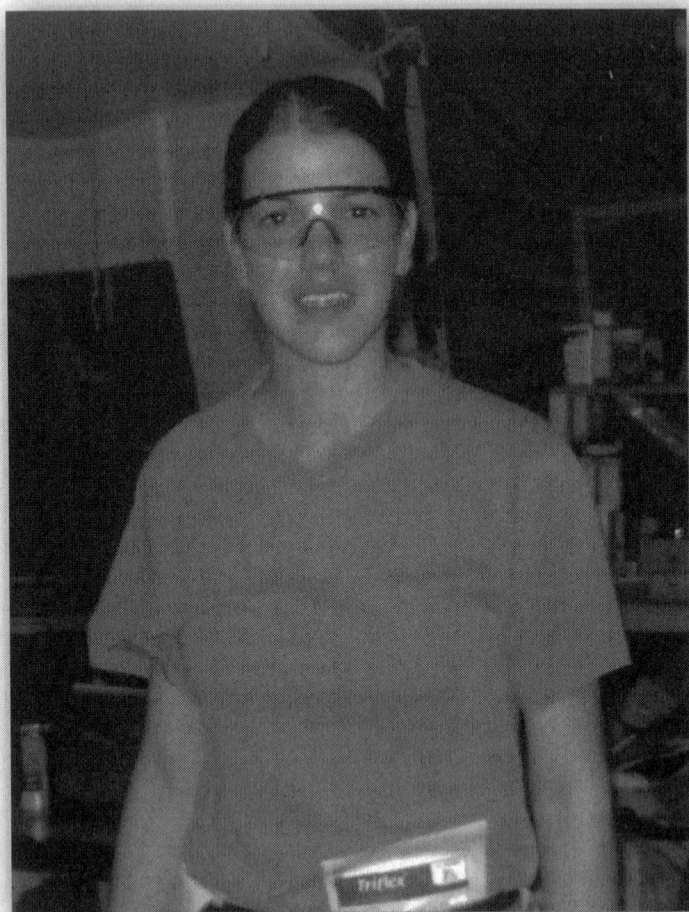

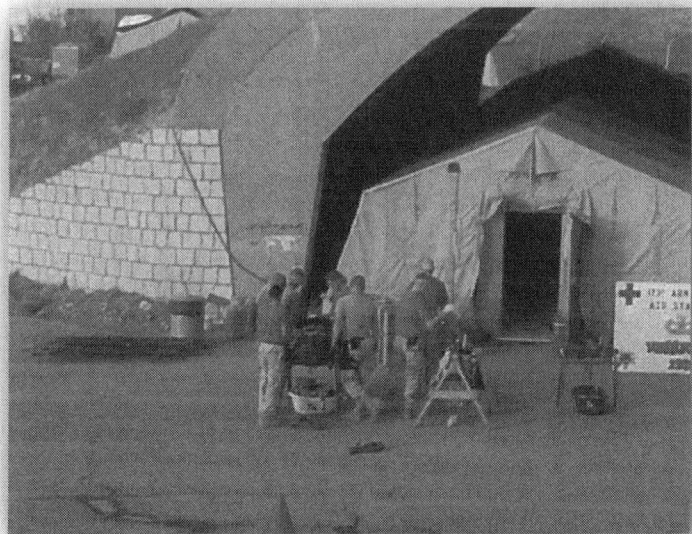

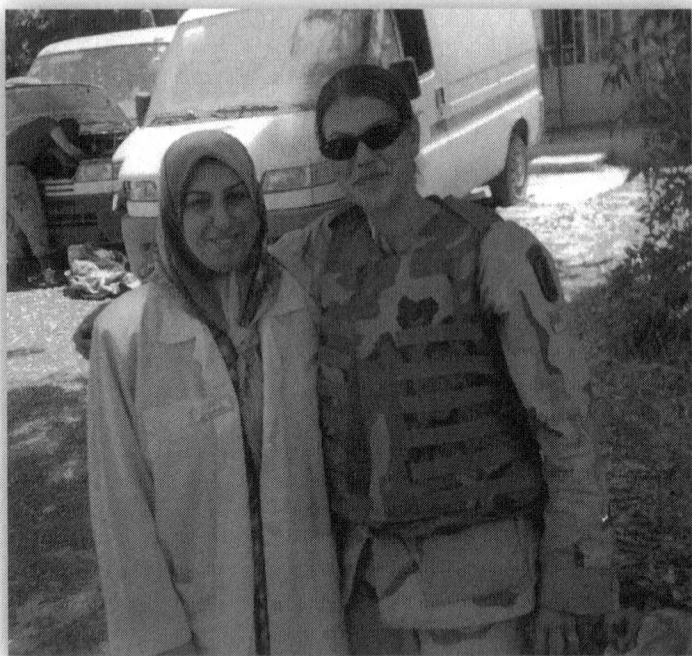

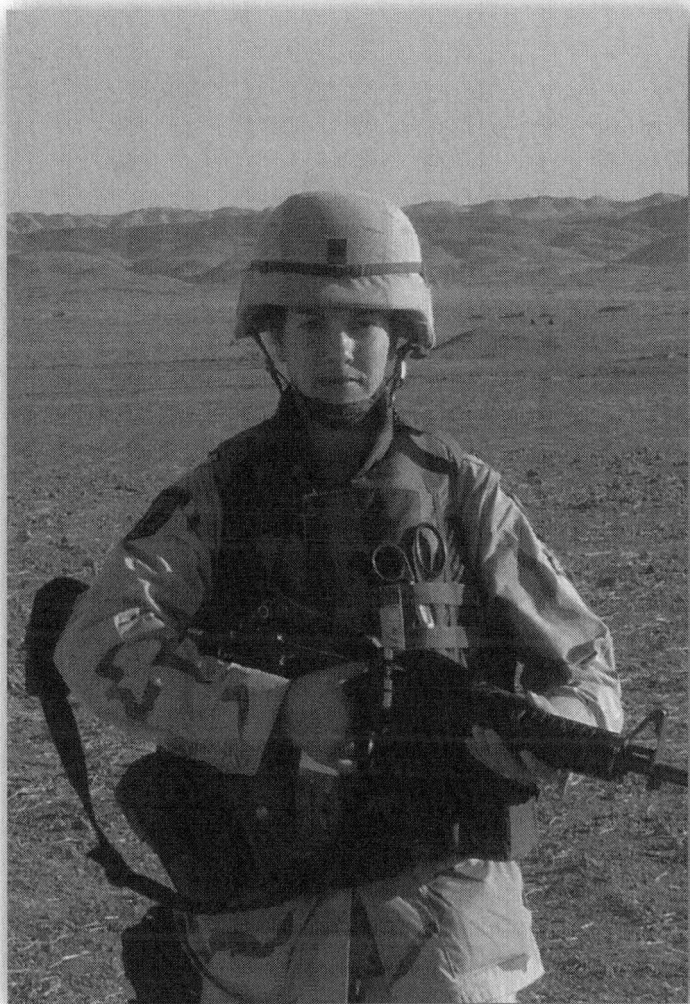

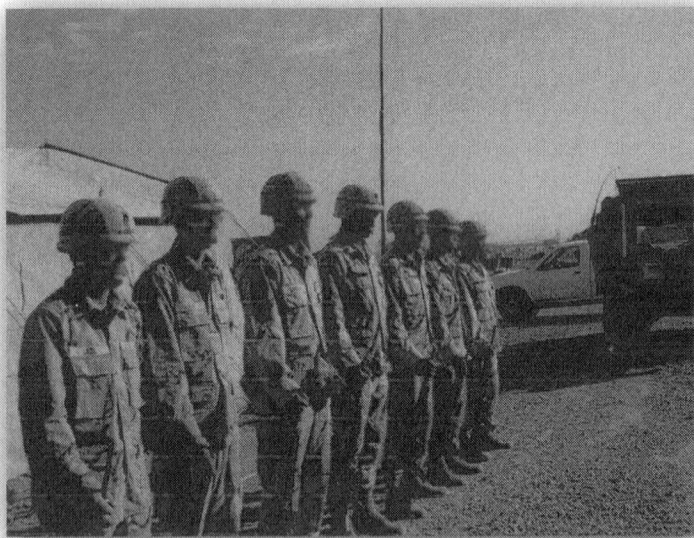

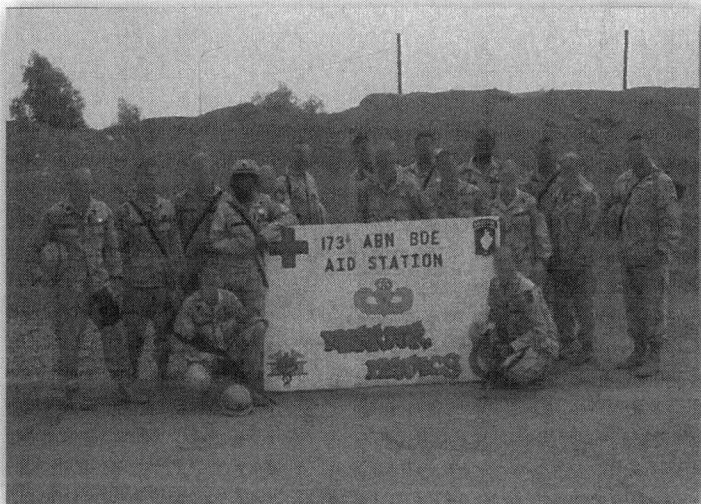

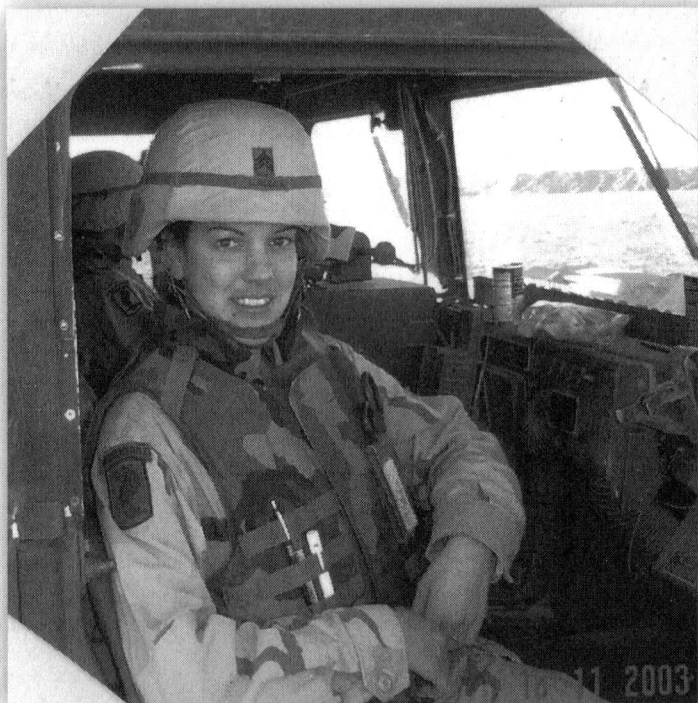

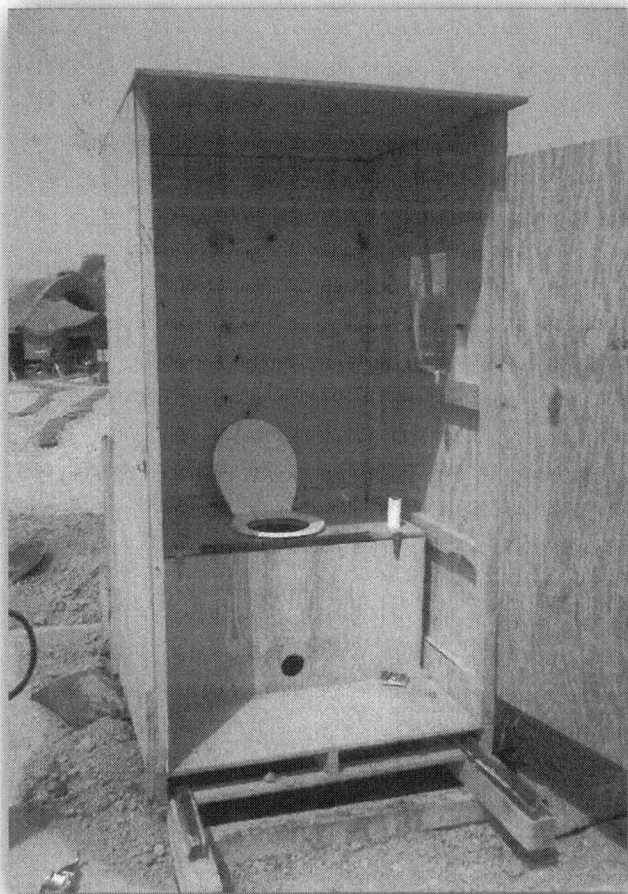

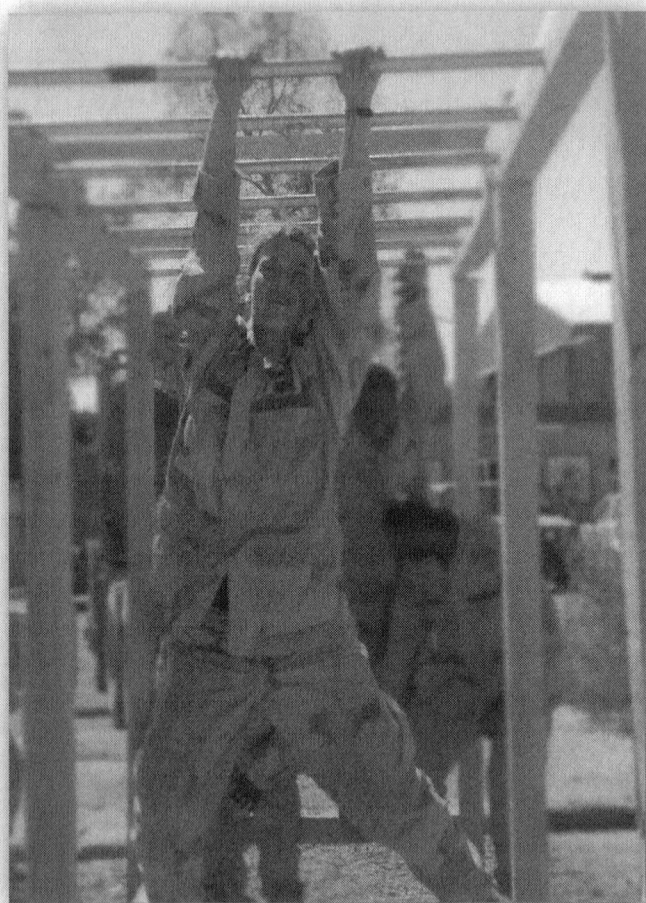

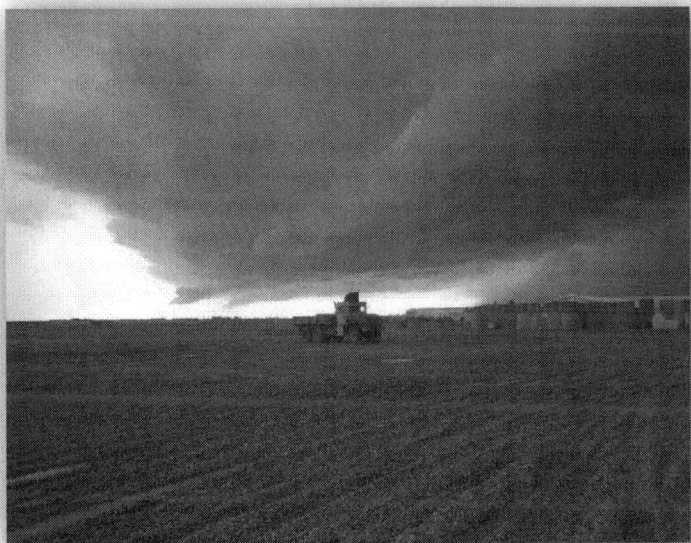

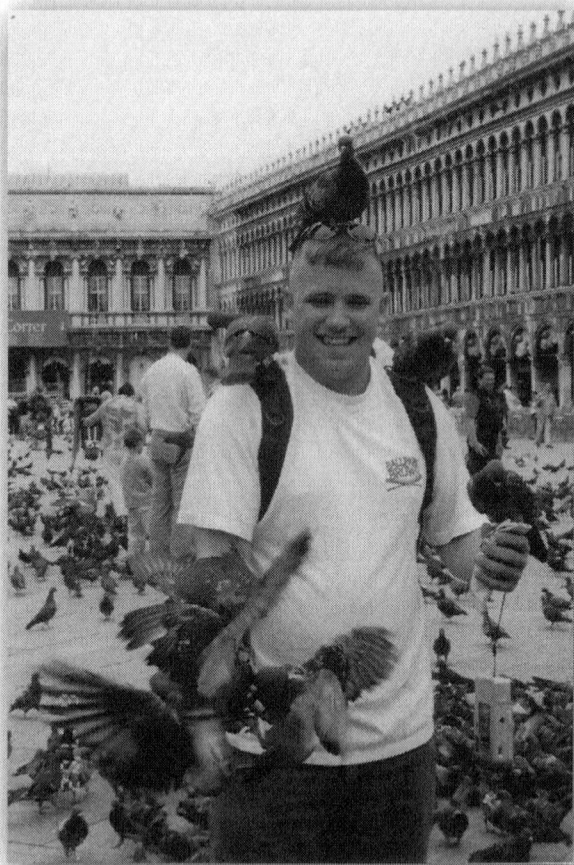

Sergeant Michael Yashinski

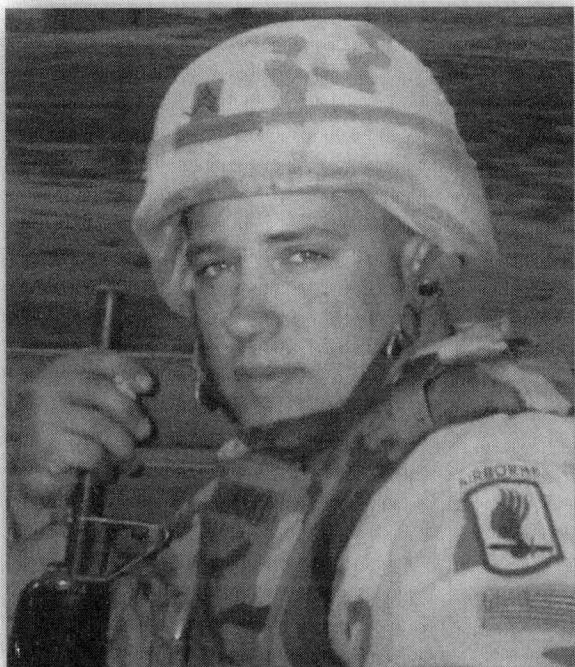

Sergeant Michael Yashinski

Statement from his mother: "Michael, you are my buddy, my heart, my life. Your dad and I will miss you always, until we meet again."

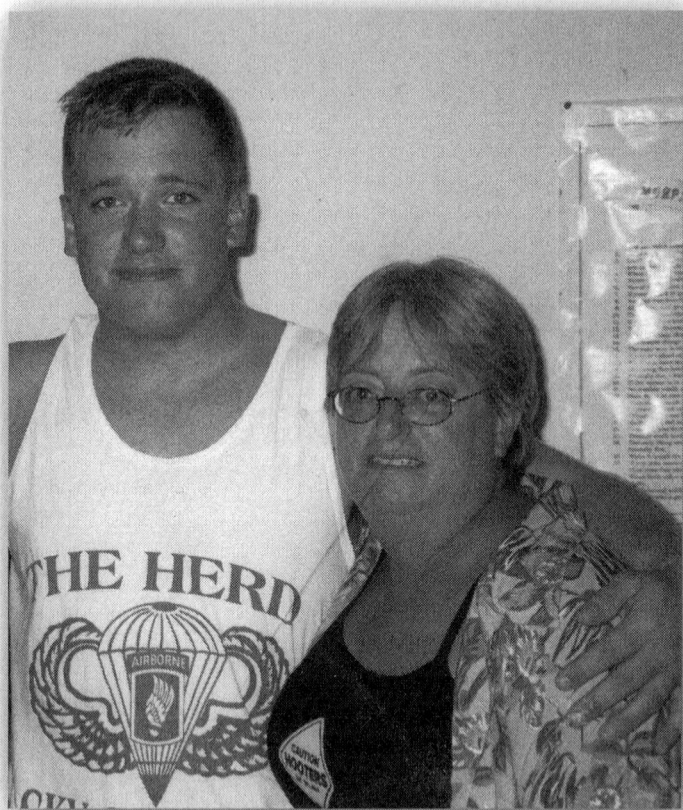

Sergeant Yashinski and his mother Deb

THE CHAOTIC MESS

CIVILIANS ON THE battlefield were almost the hardest to treat. We saw them regularly in the aid station probably due to the fact they didn't wear body armor and weren't authorized to carry a weapon.

I say they were hard because I think a lot of the time they didn't understand why this happened to them. I want to say they felt invincible sometimes. From talking to the civilian contractors, I realized that some of them really did want to carry weapons and wear body armor. This just wasn't part of their deal. Some were angry, others didn't care so much.

"Six vehicle rollover, hostile fire indicated," came over the radio. They were simply stating that they were on their way with a lot of casualties, by ground. They hadn't been

touched by any medical assets at all yet, so they were coming just as they were, open wounds and all.

We pulled out almost every bit of equipment we had
out. We were ready for these guys. In what seemed like a
short minute, three white SUVs swung around the corner
at top speed. The next three vehicles were civilian trucks.
The SUVs had noticeable damage. The windows were shattered, and blood was smeared everywhere.

Every medic in sight ran up to one of the six trucks. We
had to do a triage and determined who had the worst injury
so we could prioritize who could be treated first. This was
extremely difficult due to the fact that there were people
and medics and doctors and trucks spread all over the place.
It was pure *chaos*.

The first guy I saw was holding his head in his hands.
He was in the front passenger seat, and the windshield in
front of him was shattered to pieces. There was blood all
over the place. I yelled for a litter. We got the guy into the
aid station, and I handed him over to an NCO (noncommissioned officer) that was in there waiting to man a table.

The next guy was really bad off. He had been shot. The
bullet had traveled into his thigh and through his right tes-
ticle. He was bleeding profusely from his femoral artery.
We had to suppress the bleeding and get him out of there
fast. In a quick five minutes, he had covered the entire work
area beneath us with blood. He was drifting in and out of
consciousness. He had no idea who he was or what had

happened, but within the golden ten minutes, he was on a bird and out of sight.

The casualty I then worked on was an American contractor in his mid-forties, around my father's age at the time. He had cuts and scrapes all over him, requiring numerous amounts of stitches. I grabbed some of the other medics who had already treated and evacuated their casualties. This guy seemed to have only minor cuts and scrapes at first. The doctor told me to start sewing the long cut on his forehead. I noticed this man seemed rather sleepy and not in a whole lot of pain. That was a bit peculiar to me.

I rechecked his head, and when my fingers ran over the back of his head, I felt something strange. It felt like a loose piece of skin. I didn't want to roll him over for fear of a spinal injury, so I grabbed another medic to help me lift his head up a little.

When we did, I was astonished to what I saw. The back of his scalp was split wide open into an avulsion, but the cut across his head was so clean the flap of skin laid perfectly pressed and sealed with blood to his head. I called the doc over and showed him. He told me to put some sterile gloves on and that we were "going in." I didn't like that term at all.

I came back with sterile gloves on, and Doc Jacobs grabbed my hand and rubbed my finger under this man's scalp and into the bone. It felt so weird. I felt this man's skull and the piece of his scalp that was trying to cover it. When I pulled my hand out, I noticed what looked like brain matter on my fingers. I couldn't be sure, but that's what it looked like. I almost got sick. Then the doc asked me to do something I wasn't sure I would be able to handle. I had to irrigate this wound out, which meant have someone lift the flap of scalp, and with pressure squeeze these bottles of sterile water into his head. My pulse was racing, and sweat was building up and streaming down my face.

The irrigating was by far the worst of it. A pasty red color mix came spurting out of his head with the water. I irrigated until it was clear. Then I spent about fifteen minutes stitching up his scalp. In the meantime, other medics were talking to this man, keeping him awake. I feared he would die in our care. That is the worst fear for a medic.

Once we were done, he was evacuated to Germany. I said a silent prayer for this man to survive. I prayed to God he would make it home to his family.

JOSE

BILLY (MY THEN fiancé) was in a ranger unit within our brigade. They were always out on high-speed missions and patrols. They are elite so are often picked to conduct dangerous duties. His good friend Jose Banuelos (Banjo) was in his platoon. Billy and I had been together for about two years at the time, and I knew his buddies well. Jose was the one whom I knew like a brother. He was always looking out for me. He even called me "sis."

The day Jose got shot was a day like no other. I was prepared for anything, but not this. I knew when the call came over the radio that some LRS soldiers had been hurt; chances were I knew who it was. I waited impatiently inside the treatment tent. I wanted to be on a table. When I saw Jose, my first reaction was disbelief. *No way,* I thought. "B (I called him), what the hell happened?" his voice was as calm as ever. You would have never thought this guy was shot in the femur four times! "Liss, it's all right, dude. Please don't be upset, sis." He was so sincere and cared so much about how I felt. I was just holding his hand and hugging him, almost forgetting I was a medic with a job to do.

Jose began telling me the story. He was riding in a Nissan patrol SUV, conducting a convoy for a simple mission. They left the "safe house" (a house that is guarded by our own) and went about a normal patrol out in the town.

All of a sudden, they heard gunfire. Jose doesn't remember even firing back; it was all so sudden. They were hit with an RPG (rocket-propelled grenade) followed by some machine-gun action. They say the enemy was on higher ground so they had that leeway. Jose was struck while riding in the truck trying to pass up the ambush.

He spent less than half an hour with us before he was ready to go to the Air Force. He had four bullets in his leg according to our x-rays. They were beyond the point where we could take them out. This had to be surgically done.

I went the next day to visit him hearing that he was flying out to Germany soon. I wanted to say good-bye because he probably was out of the war for good. I walked in to find him being spoiled by the Air Force nurses. Pretty ones too! He was being well taken care of. I brought him some magazines and a soda from the chow hall. Jose grabbed my hand and pulled me into a hug. "Thanks, Liss." I was in tears at this point. I looked at his leg, and it was pulled tautly into this metal splint that was screwed into his leg. It looked painful, but he said he didn't feel it. They had him pretty drugged up. I said good-bye to him. I wouldn't see him for almost six months later.

Jose eventually made it home and took one of the bullets from his leg that they had given him, had it bronzed, and made it into a necklace. He went home on convalescent leave to sunny California. He wrote me letters from home explaining how nice it was there, but always mentioned he would rather be back in Iraq with his troops in the thick of it.

I wanted to see Billy. This was, after all, his friend first. Billy had just left Iraq on orders to Florida's 6th Ranger Training Battalion to be a ranger instructor. I was sad he was gone and knew I would have to tell him the story over the phone—something I was not looking forward to. I called him that night and told him the news. He was so upset he wasn't there with his guys. I felt for him. I knew how badly he still wanted to be there, not just for me but also for guys like Jose. I selfishly just wanted him there to come and see me and to take away all my worry and emotional pain. I knew I wouldn't see him or Jose for at least six months.

THANKSGIVING

THE HOLIDAYS WERE difficult in Iraq.

The Fourth of July I landed my feet in the desert, then on my birthday I was involved in the IED attack, and now it was Thanksgiving—the time to give thanks to all God has allowed us to have and cherish. We all took some part in preparation for the big dinner.

Some of us decorated, others helped cook, and I helped on the grill. The dinner turned out beautiful. The food was delicious and the decorations were amazing. I must have taken twenty pictures at dinner. My prayer before dinner was, "Thank you, Lord, for the safety you have bestowed upon all of us. Thank you for taking care of the wounded and for guiding the deceased through your path and to heaven. Thank you, Lord, for this wonderful meal, and we pray to all get home safe and sound. In Jesus's name I pray, amen."

It seemed as though bad things always happened on significant dates, so we were all armed with small Motorola radios while at the chow hall. Amazingly enough throughout dinner, the radios remained silent, but we were all paranoid. We usually left one medic and the radio guard at the aid station.

Toward the end of our dinner, when we were all gathering around for pictures for our families, that call finally came over the radio. "We got a nine-line coming in.". *Great*, I thought. *Here we go again.*

My platoon grabbed the last of their food and shoved it down on the way out. Time to get our game faces on. We all hauled butt back to the aid station, which was about on thousand meters away from the chow hall.

The birds had already lifted off and were ten minutes out. The casualties we had coming in were involved in a raid, and some had gunshot wounds.

Before we knew it, the choppers had landed, and the FLA was off to pick them up. My squad leader was not around, so I took charge of my team. I placed one medic in charge of taking vital signs, one medic to write the SOAP note (subjective, objective, assessment, and plan). Another medic was to initiate the IV (intravenous infusion) and was responsible for pushing medications such as morphine. The last medic on my team was to be the irrigator. I told them all to remove their DCU (Desert Combat Uniform) tops and just remain in their tan T-shirts. "Let's get gloved up."

We were far more ready than ever before when they arrived. It seemed like our reaction time got better every time, which only made sense since we were having so much practice.

"Okay, guys, it's Thanksgiving and our bellies are full. Let's be on our toes. These guys probably didn't get turkey today."

The first casualty was a small infantryman. He was maybe nineteen years old. He was alert and oriented but had a nice gunshot wound to his arm.

The next was a medic in the infantry unit. Most of us knew him, so it was difficult. He had a large piece of shrapnel from a blast that was lodged behind his right shoulder. It was a very large impalement. There wasn't a whole lot we could do for him because it probably involved several nerves and arteries. We could only wrap it in place and get him the hell out of there.

Two more guys came in. They were with the same infantry unit. One was out of it and had a gunshot wound to his neck. It was bleeding profusely. He was sent directly to the Forward Surgical Team, which worked in conjunction with us. They were just five hundred meters away on the other side. We would always send casualties there who required immediate life-saving surgery. They were a huge help.

The other guy was another gunshot wound. He had been shot in the thigh and was cussing up a storm. My team was working on him, and he would not calm down. I told him in order for us to treat him the best way we can, he's going to have to try and calm down. He did so, and we were able to get some information out of him. The GSW (gunshot wound) did not go all the way through his leg, so it was actually still in there. The doctor came over and told us it was at our level, that we could do this.

I applied some sterile gloves, and Doc Jacobs came over to assist me and provide me guidance in removing the bullet. I never thought I would be sitting here removing a bullet out of someone's leg. It was crazy. *This poor kid*, I thought.

It only took maybe fifteen minutes, and we had it out. Surprisingly enough, the bullet was not in his leg that deep, maybe a half inch. I snatched some of my guys to take turns in stitching his leg up. They did an excellent job.

These casualties stayed with us for a few nights. The evacuation out of theatre was getting backed up now, and they were required to stay longer, awaiting transportation. This only meant we were getting busier. I would go into the patient-hold tent at night and chat with some of the patients. Sometimes they would just lie there and stare at the tent ceiling as if reminiscing about home or thinking of the horrors of war. Regardless, I just wanted to cheer them up. Civilians and soldiers alike, they needed someone—anyone—who cared to be by their side. Medics in my platoon were always good about keeping the casualties company until it was their time to leave.

A CHRISTMAS TRAGEDY

WE WERE ALL pumped up about Christmas. It was only two days away, and some soldiers had all their gifts from their families piled up next to their cots. Mine were all wrapped inside their cardboard boxes. I had about seven cards that I had not yet opened. I made myself wait until Christmas Day. It just seemed the traditional thing to do. I have a very supportive family. My parents and brothers were all very consistent about keeping me up on all the current magazines, snacks, and waterless shampoos.

I was sometimes placed in charge of coordinating the barbeques or parties that we would have to boost our morale. This one I was put in charge of was, of course, a Christmas party. It was to be on Christmas Eve because our chow hall was going to have a big Christmas dinner on Christmas Day.

Everyone was giving me decorations that they had received from their families in the mail. I was sent a small Christmas tree and some decorations. I put that on the center table in the classroom that our combat support engineer company helped us build when we first moved locations.

My buddy Kati helped me string up the decorations and place all the cakes and cookies out that people donated. Then it was time to start cooking the meat. We went to the chow hall, and they gave us some steaks and side items. I was in charge of the beans because I'm not much of a grill master.

One of our physician assistants, Captain Monti, was really into the grill. He and a fellow medic, Specialist Cipolla, enjoyed seasoning and cooking the steaks to perfection. We all took pride in our own areas.

I brought my little radio out and put some Christmas music on. It had started to get dark, so some soldiers brought the spotlight over. We got a hold of some eggnog and sipped on it while we were cooking. Even though there was no snow on the ground and the temperatures were sitting at eighty degrees in December, the spirit of Christmas was definitely in the air.

Just as we were all laughing about some joke Kati had made, this guy in another platoon came frantically running over to us. He was yelling something but at first we couldn't make out what he was saying. Then it dawned on me. He was yelling that someone had been electrocuted and was laid out on the pavement.

Oh my God, on Christmas Eve, I thought.

That person turned out to be Sergeant Michael Yashinski (or Sergeant Ski, as we all knew him). He was our communications specialist. He dealt with us all the time. We constantly had problems with our radios, or telephones, or Internet. He was over all the time fixing something. I had known SGT Yashinski for a couple of years in the unit. I knew he was so excited as he was to be out of the Army in only a few short months.

I wondered why they brought him directly to the Forward Surgical Team. I couldn't understand why he didn't come to us instead. As our physician assistant and another medic ran over to the FST to help out, I was told what had happened.

He was up on a ladder about twenty-five feet off the ground. He was trying to fix something with the live wires and was shocked. The shock sent him flying all twenty-five feet down to the pavement. They said he landed flat on his face and when they rolled him over, he was unconscious. The words I heard were, "He looked dead." No. I refused to believe it. They're going to save him, I know it. I had utter faith and confidence in the Forward Surgical Team. They proved so many times they can perform miracles, even if someone is unconscious.

We still had meat on the grill and beans in the bowls. It was difficult to understand how or what we should be doing. I talked with Kati about going over there to help. There were too many people over there already, she said. So all we could do was wait, and it was killing me. I had to know something.

It was a good twenty minutes before we saw the PA and one of our medics walking slowly in our direction. I could tell from the looks on their faces this was not good.

"What happened? How is he?"

They simply shook their heads in disbelief.

"There was nothing we could do. He was already gone."

Oh my God, this can't be happening. It's Christmas Eve!

I knew the Army had to tell the next of kin within twenty-four hours and that it would probably be Christmas Day when they found out their twenty-four-year-old son, who was three months from being a civilian, was dead.

We were all in complete and utter shock. Just like that and someone can be gone forever. I had no words, no thoughts, just sorrow. I was in disbelief. Needless to say, my appetite had vanished, and it just didn't seem so jolly anymore. I went to sleep that night knowing that the next day—Christmas Day—someone was going to knock on his parent's door and tell them their son was gone…forever.

BIOGRAPHY OF MICHAEL EMERSON YASHINSKI

(Courtesy of Debora Yashinski)

Michael Emerson Yashinski was born on October 8, 1979, in Camp Lejeune, NC. He was the son of Marine SSGT Jim and Debbie Yashinski. He was their one and only son. Michael lived at many bases until he was in the second grade. His family then moved to Colorado and Michael graduated from Lewis Palmer High School in 1997. Michael was an athlete. He played baseball, football, wrestling, and hockey (hockey being his favorite). He was a champion tomahawk and knife thrower. He loved black powder shooting and had a percussion .50 caliber Kentucky long rifle.

Michael had wanted to join the military since he was young. His father, grandfather, and uncle were all marines, but Michael joined the Army to go airborne.

His mother recalls the excitement in his voice after he made his first parachute jump. "He called me and said, 'mom, it is so peaceful and quiet. It's like looking into the face of God'."

Michael was trained in communications and upon airborne school completion, he was assigned to Fort Bragg, NC. He served his time at Fort Bragg and in 2001 was sent to Vicenza, Italy, to join the 173rd Airborne Brigade, 501st Forward Support Company, Headquarters Platoon. He loved his job, Italy, and the Italians. He made many friends. He deployed with the 173rd in March 2003. While in Iraq, he would call home and tell his mom not to worry, everything was okay. Michael was devastated in August of 2003 when fellow 501st soldier and friend Craig Ivory died from a stroke. He had asked his mom to do a memorial drawing in memory of Craig. She did a drawing of a kneeling soldier with fallen ID tags. She had no idea one day she'd be adding her own son's ID tags to the drawing. Michael is described by his family as loyal, honest, loving, supportive, intelligent, and funny. Just turned twenty-four, Michael died doing the job that he loved. He was fixing some live wires for the company when he was electrocuted on Christmas Eve 2003.

Michael is survived by his mother, father, grandfather, aunt and uncle, and cousins.

NEW YEAR'S BREAK

DURING OUR TOUR in Iraq, some of the soldiers were allowed to fly back to the states for what is called R & R, or "rest and relaxation." It was a good program. It gave them time to recuperate and spend time with their families. Some soldiers had pregnant wives or brand-new babies or sick relatives whom they needed to see.

I had only been in Iraq since the Fourth of July, as my comrades had been there since the war began—March 25. The New Year was approaching, and I knew there was a four-day R & R trip to the country of Qatar. They sent soldiers on the four-day trips if they had been in country a shorter period of time and were not on the list to go back to the states. My friend Kati had only been there since August, so neither one of us was allowed to take leave to go to the States. We asked to go on this trip to Qatar, which fell over the New Year holiday.

They told us later that we were to be on this bus that next morning at 0500 hours. We threw the one pair of civilian clothes we had brought and our bath articles into our backpacks. I grabbed my digital camera knowing this would make for some interesting pictures for my family.

That next day was the 30th of December. Instead of taking this bus, they loaded us up on a CH-47 Chinook helicopter. It was an amazing flight. We got to see all of Iraq and the mountains leading into Qatar. It was beautiful. I just sat there and thought about how we were able to leave all the drama for a few days. I was so excited.

When we arrived, they showed us to our bays where we would be sleeping. We stayed in this hanger that had separate male and female bays with rows and rows of bunk beds. It was close to the way I lived in basic training.

The first night we were there, we took the first real shower we had had in months. It was wonderful. I could have stayed in there all night and been completely content. The water was hot and the pressure was great. I couldn't believe how much I had missed this.

We left the hanger and walked to this little pub on the camp. It was like an officer's club. All the people there were on the same type R & R that we were. Some soldiers we talked to were out of Iraq, Afghanistan, and Kuwait. It was neat because everyone had his or her own stories. I was not particularly fond of sharing mine.

We found out we were allowed to drink alcohol here, which was forbidden in Iraq. They gave us a three-beer limit. I had no idea how much my tolerance had changed until I finished that first beer. It was a German beer so it had higher alcohol content. As hard as I tried, I could not stop thinking about Iraq. I wanted to know what my fellow medics were doing. I felt guilty in a way for being here when some of my guys were still out there.

We relaxed and socialized with groups of people from all over the place. It was difficult to not get depressed a little, especially with the alcohol kicking in. I only had two that night and felt like just going to sleep.

The next day we went to the PX on the camp and bought some civilian clothes. Then we ate at the Chili's restaurant they had on post. I was so excited to have real food. I hadn't had any decent food, except for on holidays, so I was ready for this tasty meal. It was so good. I ate so fast I got heartburn. I couldn't believe how awesome this food was.

Between the shower, the bed, and the real food, it made me realize how much we take for granted in every day life. We don't realize there are people out there who live the way we do in Iraq, but every day of their lives.

I slept wonderful that night.

The next morning, Kati and I journeyed over to the hanger where you can sign up for certain trips. They picked our names out of the hat for the desert safari trip. It sounded neat. I had no idea what we were in store for.

We showed up on our scheduled time with a group of about twenty-five soldiers. These Arab men with turbans on their heads picked us up in about seven SUVs with dark tinted windows. I was a little nervous riding somewhere in the middle of the desert with these guys.

We took off and drove on the highway for about twenty minutes before we reached the dirt turn off. They changed something on the gears and we slowed down quite a bit. Before I knew it, we were practically buried in this soft sand.

After driving for about five minutes into the desert, I realized we couldn't see anything else. It was like the rest of the country had dropped off the face of the planet. We were surrounded by berms of beautiful cream-colored sand. It was amazing. It reminded me of a postcard I once saw on the Sahara Desert.

I held my camera out the window to snap some pictures. It was like nothing I had ever seen before. I couldn't believe we were in this beautiful place when two days earlier we were staring at blood. It was truly a deserved break.

The Arab men made a stop for us to take pictures. We stopped at the top of this berm and we were overlooking the water. It was gorgeous. Kati and I walked to the edge and looked at the blue-green crystal-clear water. We took a lot of pictures and then played in the sand. It was so fine, almost like salt. I had never felt sand like that before. You could scoop a handful up, and it would just seep through your fingertips like water.

We climbed back in the trucks and headed out on the trail. The drivers started to pick up speed now. We went down and around these mountains of flowing sand. You could see creases in the hills as if the sand just wouldn't stop flowing. It was amazing.

The next stop we made was sudden. We went around this hill, and it opened up into a large barbeque site. There were Arabs out there cooking on the grill. There were plastic tables set up with tiki torches. There was a tent that had cushions on the floor for sitting and a gigantic Arab rug in the center. It was very festive and overlooking the beach.

We all got out and took our shoes off to walk through the sand. It felt so wonderful beneath my toes. We were to be here for a couple of hours. We went down to the beach and rolled up our jeans. Walking through the clear water, I realized how amazing this place was. I had never seen anything like this before. I felt as if I didn't even deserve this. I had a mission to do, and I felt guilty for being in this gorgeous relaxing place.

The food they grilled for us was very good. We couldn't tell what some things were, and I even had the notion they might be poisoning us. I had to tell myself this was an Army function and they were Arab, not Iraqi enemies.

It was time to go back to the camp now, and we knew the next day we would be heading back to Iraq. I was sad and happy all at the same time. I felt as though this break was truly needed, but I was ready to continue the mission in

Iraq. We only had a couple of months left. I could toughen it out. We loaded the buses the next day, and it was back to reality.

THE FIRST MORTAR ATTACK

AFTER THE NICE break in Qatar, I knew something bad was bound to happen. It was kind of like the holidays. Every holiday we had a nervous feeling, and they usually proved to be correct.

On this particular day, it was rather quiet. Work seemed to be flowing as normal. The regular day-to-day sick patients would come in and be seen, and then sent on their way. We had a regular welcome, "Hey, welcome back, time to get to work!" Business as usual.

It started to get dark outside as I was smoking a ciga-rette. This was a habit of mine that I grew particularly fond of during the deployment. It seemed to be my sense of freedom for the time being. I would go outside and sit down somewhere, smoke, and stare up at the stars. I would think about what my family was doing and how the rest of the world was taking what must have been horrifying news on Iraq.

I enjoyed my last smoke for the night and was heading to my living area for some shut-eye. I had only been in my sleep tent for a few minutes when the first one flew over us. It was a very certain whistling sound. I knew it was something bad. This was the first mortar round I had actually heard in person. My whole body froze. In this type of situation that we had trained for, we would all grab our body armor and run for the bunker—but it was different when it actually happened. I froze, and so did everyone else in the tent. My mind wanted to run and tell everyone to run to the bunker, but my body wouldn't let me move.

Kati was cleaning up the patient-holding tent, as she was on the night shift. She stuck her head in the tent entrance and quietly said, "I think that was a mortar round and we just got hit!"

I immediately snapped out of my temporary coma and started yelling at the soldiers in the tent.

"All right, you all know the drill. Grab your gear and get in the bunker now!"

People were frantic. It was chaotic. I knew we were being attacked. The whistling sound was just that. It was only a second or two after we heard the whistling that we heard the impact. It was a loud and dull landing, but I was praying it was a dud.

As my troops gathered their gear and started running out of the tent, another mortar round flew over us. I came outside after everyone else was out and headed for the bunker. The sky lit up like it was the Fourth of July. There were bright red tracers coming over my head from every direction. I heard several blasts, whistling, and lots of people yelling.

The Air Force came over the loud speaker they had set up in the center of the camp: "ALARM RED! ALARM RED! All personnel, don your body armor and seek immediate shelter. ALARM RED!"

This went on over and over for several minutes. It was so loud you could still hear it from inside the bunker. Whenever an attack was over, they would come back on and call ALARM GREEN.

It was close to five minutes after the initial mortar round hit when we had accountability of all soldiers. There were even a few soldiers who were at the gym on camp working out at the time of the attack. They were back in minutes. It was a very quick reaction time. I was pleased, along with the rest of the team.

That night no one was hurt by the mortar attack. We were lucky that time. God was surely on our side. We later found out that one of the rounds had landed on the backside of the gym, next to a port-a-potty. It *was* a dud.

I prayed and thanked God for that because there would have been so many traumas had that gym been hit. Another one hit directly on the airfield, and the third landed outside of our camp. They had missed their target. We had defeated them.

The mortar attacks came every now and again. They were conducting target practice. Every time they would get closer and closer to our post. Our camp was eventually hit and damaged, but it was long after we were gone. That was one of the scariest nights of my life—my first mortar attack.

TROUBLE IN PARADISE

FOR A WHILE, I thought things could not get any worse. Boy, was I wrong!

One of my soldiers, PFC Blake, had been pulling gate guard on the front gate of the camp for a month or so. He came in the tent one day and told me he had some packages he had to send. So I signed out a Humvee with the soldier on radio watch and took him to the camp's post office.

We stood in line for almost an hour. People were constantly sending home things like Iraqi carpets, pictures, cameras, and Christmas gifts they didn't need just yet. Blake had five boxes to send home that he said he didn't have time to do during the holidays.

A civilian woman working there was checking through all the boxes to find things you weren't allowed to send home. An Iraqi bayonet was surely one of those things.

Blake pulled this bayonet out of one of his packages and held it up. "Can I send this?" he asked. The lady just glared at him and replied *no*, so he put it in his pocket. I gave him a nudge telling him he should have known that. I felt like maybe I hadn't emphasized that when I put the information out to the soldiers.

When we turned around to leave, I saw the brigade sergeant major standing there shaking his head. I could only say, "I know, Sergeant Major." And then we left.

The next day, my platoon sergeant came in our tent screaming. I jumped up and went to see what the problem was.

"Sergeant Lonsdale, get outside now!" he yelled.

I hurried outside to find the whole platoon out there in formation.

I was thinking I had missed a timeline or something because I was the only one in the tent. That was not the case. He had this whole thing planned.

Staff Sergeant (SSG) Miller began, "Now, we all know what we can and can't send home right? Because apparently some of us were confused. Blake, being Sergeant Lonsdale's soldier, decided he wanted to try and send an Iraqi bayonet home through the mail. Sergeant Lonsdale, being the NCO, should have informed her soldier that he was not authorized to send it. So here's what we're going to do. All the sergeants standing out here will go gather all their gear and lay it out here dress right dress. The soldiers will stand by to inspect. You all have five minutes. Go!"

I was shocked. How did he find out about that? Then I remembered that the sergeant major was standing behind us. He has meetings every night with all the company's first sergeants. Our first sergeant must have told SSG Miller this morning. I still thought they blew the whole thing out of proportion.

We laid all of our gear outside dress right dress so that it was all matching each other's. Then he had the soldiers call off items from the list and hold up our stuff. For one, it was embarrassing because I knew from my soldier's mistake that it was unintentionally my fault. I felt like everyone was upset with me.

After the layout, all the sergeants in formation had to recite the noncommisioned officer (NCO) creed in front of the platoon. Some of them messed up the words. I had no problem because I had just finished the basic noncommissioned officer's course in which we had to recite the creed three times a day.

Once we were dismissed from the formation, I went back to my sleep area to put my stuff away. I thought that was the end of it. I was wrong. SSG Miller called me outside and told me I was to meet him in the classroom at 2100 (9 p.m.) for my counseling statement.

In the Army, if you do something wrong, they will give you a counseling statement. This is a form that states what you did, and what we can do to fix it, or corrective training. I dreaded what that was going to be.

I met him in the classroom, and he proceeded to read the counseling statement to me. Although I didn't agree with the way things were worded, I signed it anyway. Then he told me "For your corrective training, Sergeant, you are hereby assigned to guard the front gate indefinitely."

I couldn't believe it. I almost started crying. I did not want to leave my soldiers. I was running a squad and begged and pleaded for him to come up with something else. "Please, Sergeant. I can't leave my soldiers for the rest of the time we're here."

He replied with, "Well, you obviously weren't doing a very good job, were you?"

So that was it. I was off to guard the front gate of the post until it was time for us to go. My showtime was five in the morning. I walked out upset. I went right to my cot to get my gear ready.

GUARDING THE GATES

I FIGURED THIS was going to be hell on earth. I couldn't stand the thought of standing there all day staring at a gate and checking passes while my soldiers patched up broken paratroopers. My stomach ached for them.

A Sergeant First Class Neuman picked me up in a white SUV. He seemed very nice. He was the platoon sergeant for our combat support company (engineers). He told me he was the noncommissioned officer in charge of all the gates. I was to be in charge of gate 5. This was the gate that allowed a lot of the Iraqis who had construction contracts to come on post. I realized I was going to be "in charge" and not just a guard. This was better than I thought.

We got to the gate, and I saw a few people on the detail whom I knew. It was good because we would be out here all day every day, and I wanted to have people around me whom I could converse with.

It was actually starting to get chilly outside, even with the sunlight. I jumped out of the truck and threw on my body armor, which I was to wear at all times while manning the gate. This was going to take some getting used to. We never wore the body armor at the aid station unless we were being attacked and had to run into the bunkers, or if we went outside the camp on a mission.

The first person I saw was SGT John Nelson. He was a friend of mine whom I had gotten to know while we trained in places like Germany and Hungary. John was a nice guy and very funny. I knew he would make this experience somewhat enjoyable. He gave me the very brief tour of the gate and explained our duties while on the gate.

I was put in charge of this gate and was given one of the two SUVs that we had to man the gates. SFC Neuman had the other one. He said he would pop in occasionally to check up on things. I was grateful to have my own truck but shocked at what I found when I opened the door. It was a stick shift! I never drove a stick shift before. There was a point in my teenage years when my father tried to teach me, but after almost running his truck into my school, he got frustrated. We went out and bought an automatic.

So it had been a good nine years since I had even attempted to drive a standard vehicle. All the trucks in the Army that I was licensed on were automatic. I knew I had to learn how to drive this truck in a timely manner.

SGT Nelson quickly took on the task of instructing me. It took about three days for me to grasp the idea of the clutch and the gas at the same time. I stalled out about ten times a day at first. Then I was finally ready to put it in third gear. The "escorts" (soldiers who guarded the contractors) all rode around with me in the mornings to chow, to work, and then at the end of the day back to their tents.

They got a kick out of seeing this *Sergeant* attempt to drive a standard SUV. This was the joke of the day usually. It wasn't long before I had it down, and it was actually enjoyable.

John was my right-hand man. He was my "runner" on the gate. Whatever was needed, I could call on him—whether it be to run and get chow for the escorts or to pick someone up whose contractor is done.

Everyone had small radios to stay in touch with another. The system went something like this: A contractor truck would show up with Iraqi workers in it. I would send one of my escorts to take the driver to pick up his badge at the main gate. They would come back and get in the truck to go to wherever the contractor's site on camp was. The soldier would sit there and watch the Iraqis work all day long. I would send Nelson to pick up chow around lunchtime, and he would bring it out to the escorts. The Iraqis brought their food with them.

Sometimes there would be a lot of downtime. The Iraqis had holidays and hardly anyone would show up. I spent a lot of those days just having conversations with John and whoever else was around. We would joke and talk about what we were going to do when we got home. We all had different visions. I saw lots of pizza. I also wanted to go to the beach and just lie around all day long. I couldn't wait to get out of this place.

The gate wasn't too stressful, but at times it could get pretty scary. I remember the bomb scare that took two hours to clear.

It was a normal day like any other—nothing out of the ordinary. Every Iraqi who came through the gate had to immediately go through a "search pit." This is where they take mirrors under the truck and let the sniffing dogs loose on the inside. They are searching for anything that can resemble something fishy. They told us when the dog sits down that something is not right. That day the dog sat.

They called over the radios for everyone to evacuate the premises. We were convinced that we had bomb in the vehicle. I was, of course, freaking out because I didn't really know how often these occurred. It took about two hours or so for the military police to clear it. When we returned, we learned that the dog had sniffed an old ammunition can that had some shell powder residue in it.

Although it was frustrating, I felt secure knowing that if the dog can smell something like that, we're pretty safe.

There were other things that worried me too though. We had a few close calls about possible car bombs. One that was called in was an orange-and-white taxicab. Well, nine out of ten cars on the streets of Iraq were orange-and-white taxicabs. This made me very nervous. We were on our toes all day. Some of the soldier escorts were infantry. They came up with a contingency plan. One guy took charge and delegated tasks to the others. They all knew where they were to stand and where to fire if that situation came to be.

Suddenly, a brown rusty-colored car came creeping up the dirt path to the gate. He drove around the concrete barriers with ease. He then stopped right in front of the gate and got out. With my M-16 pointed directly at him, I had my interpreter Ahmed ask him what his business was. He was out of gas.

I thought, *This guy is full of crap. He's pulling something fishy.* I told him to stay where he was, and then I sent one of my escorts beyond the gate to search him. With his 9-mil pointed at him, the escort patted him down and searched the car. It turned out that he really was out of gas. I was relieved, but he was still blocking traffic. Some of the soldiers volunteered to help push him out of the road, and I sent the Iraqi on foot to get some gas and return to collect his car.

Although we had many scares and call-ins, all went well on the gate. We never saw the orange-and-white taxicab that day.

THE BIG CONVOY

I WOULD GO back to my tent every night after gate guard. I was usually exhausted from the weight of the body armor and standing on my feet all day.

Some nights I would show up when the squad leaders were in meetings and I would just go to sleep. It seemed like I was an outsider at this point. I would come back and say hello to a few people and then go to sleep.

One evening, they called me back early for a briefing. I wasn't sure exactly what it was for, but I had heard a rumor we were leaving Iraq very soon. We had been waiting for our replacements for so long it seemed like they would never show up. I started to lose hope, along with everyone else. It wasn't even worth talking about anymore.

At first we were informed we would probably be flying out as a whole unit when we redeployed. Then that changed a couple of times. Now, in this meeting I had just walked into, they were talking about taking a convoy all the way down to Kuwait. Kirkuk is located in the far North of Iraq, so to get to Kuwait we would have to drive completely through Iraq—Kirkuk, Fallujah, Tikrit, Baghdad—all the bad areas. I did not believe this. I couldn't even imagine how dangerous this convoy was going to be. They were talking three days straight of driving the roads of Iraq.

I was assigned to drive our Humvee with another medic. We were to be attached to the combat support company convoy. This actually was going to work out fine. We would be one of the first convoys to leave Kirkuk. The string of convoys throughout the brigade was going to last about a week. Our scheduled departure date was the 15th of February—the day after Valentine's Day.

The time neared and we had plenty of planning to do to prepare for the long convoy to Kuwait. First I had to work on getting pulled off the gate. This was going to be a task. SSG Miller didn't see it fit to pull me off the detail until just a few days before my convoy was leaving. The medic that was supposed to ride with me, Specialist Markowitz, was attached to the long range surveillance company up until the time we were supposed to leave. So basically, I had no one there to pack up or prepare our truck for us.

I finally got pulled off gate guard about the 12th of February. Markowitz was back the next day. One hour after he returned to the aid station for good, we were heading out to the combat support company's convoy brief. This was the first of what would be many, many briefings. They were very redundant but held some good information. It was good to reiterate safety on this trip due to the fact that we had a lot of new guys who had just gotten out here.

After many briefings and drills and safety requirements, the day had finally come. February 15, 2004, we were on our way out of Iraq. I knew this was going to be one long convoy. I was glad I had Specialist Markowitz, as he was one of our most comical medics. He was always making everyone laugh with ridiculous comments and jokes. I was glad I didn't get stuck with someone boring.

We had made a plan. He would drive the first day (eight hours), I would drive the second day (fourteen hours), and he would drive into Kuwait on the third day (six hours). This was our plan, and we were going to stick to it unless one of us was falling asleep at the wheel. We had the whole setup you would normally have for a long trip—snacks, drinks, and a radio. Unfortunately we didn't have AC and couldn't do much about the extreme heat.

When we left, we were given our radio frequencies and called out in front of everyone as the "medics" on the convoy. I got that gut-wrenching feeling in my stomach again as if something bad was going to happen. I knew that if something happened within this eighteen-truck convoy, SPC Markowitz and myself would have a big mission.

We finally got onto the road about 6 a.m. There was a slight breeze in the air, and it seemed peaceful enough outside to begin our long convoy. I was nervous but yet so excited at the same time. We were finally getting out of here. I couldn't believe it was true.

We were all lined up ready to go when the officer-in-charge of the convoy approached me. "Sergeant Lonsdale, I have one extra guy who has nowhere to sit. Can he ride in the back of your truck?"

"No problem," I said and motioned for the man to jump in. *It was always good to have some added security,* I thought.

The troop's name was PFC Candon, and he seemed like a quiet guy. I just told him to pull security from the rear and that we would hook him up with snacks and things. He jumped in the back minutes before we rolled out.

The first day went by rather slow, but we had only driven five hours when we stopped for the night. I didn't understand why we were stopping for the night. We were in a town called Taji, and I found out later that this was our first day scheduled stop. We needed to stay there to regroup for the long day to follow. Markowitz and I were the thirteenth truck back in the convoy, and Nelson was the third. When we stopped, I went up to talk to him. As we were hanging out, he said, "Hey, I have something to show you."

I followed him around to the rear of his truck to find a couple of blankets balled up in the back. He asked me to look underneath. At first, I was a little hesitant because we had already seen things like gigantic camel spiders and scorpions. I slowly lifted the blankets to see two very small puppy eyes staring back at me. One was black and the other was white. They were beautiful puppies, and I almost melted with joy. He let me hold them while he talked about how they had found them wandering around near some barbwire.

He had named the white one Taji, after the town we had stopped in, and the black one was called Jihad. They were the most precious puppies I had ever seen. Even as dirty as they were, I fell in love with them.

John let me take Taji back to my vehicle for the night. We all went to our trucks to go to sleep for the night. I fell asleep under the stars on top of the hood that night snuggling with the puppy and dreaming of the day we would roll into Kuwait and out of hostile territory. It was hard to believe it was really going to happen.

The next morning, I gave Taji back to John because they had some cover on their Humvee and we didn't. The little dog could have gotten a pretty bad windburn.

Now I was in the driver's seat. I knew I had about fourteen hours to drive and was not looking forward to it, especially because we were going to be driving through Baghdad. I was nervous. I thought if anything would happen, it would be in Baghdad. They decided to take us through the off roads because going through the city would be too dangerous.

The drive became long and tedious. I daydreamed a little and thought about the little puppy a lot. I fell in love with that puppy. I couldn't wait until the next stop just to hold her again.

I felt secure with Markowitz pulling security out of the passenger-side door and Candon in the rear. I would glance back every now and then to make sure he was alert back there. The ride was going smoothly until we got a call over the radio.

The convoy that was about thirty minutes ahead of us had received direct fire. They shot back, but apparently no targets were in sight. They had just made it into Baghdad. My heart dropped. I knew two of our medics were on that convoy as well. I was fearful something bad was going to happen to our convoy when we passed through the same area. I was aware that the Iraqis knew that a large group of American soldiers were traveling far distances. I said a prayer without closing my eyes for us all to make it through Baghdad safely.

Three hours later, we were south of Baghdad, and I was relieved. I knew in my heart my prayer had something to do with it. As darkness closed in, I realized how exhausted I was. Markowitz kept asking me if I was okay to drive, and I appreciated his concern, but I had a duty and we made an agreement, so I was going to stick it out.

We made our stop that night at an Army camp south of Baghdad. It was in a pretty secure location, and I felt confident we would make it the rest of the way with no problems. We were all so exhausted and fell asleep rather quickly that night, and some of the soldiers didn't even want to make the walk to the chow hall for food. They just wanted some shut-eye.

The following day, we were motivated to go and knew by the end of the day we would be in Kuwait and officially out of Iraq. I also knew when we got into Kuwait we were going to be allowed to get rid of all of our gear. Kuwait was considered a nonhostile area, so we were pumped up about that.

We had only driven for about an hour when one of our vehicles broke down. I heard the call on the radio for the wrecker (the vehicle that carries all the towing and mechanics equipment for roadside breakdowns). The whole convoy at that point was put into a halt mode while they tried to fix the broken-down truck. We all pulled security on the left and right side of the vehicles. The rear of the convoy had some slice elements from the brigade's long range surveillance detachment. They secured the rear and stopped all incoming traffic.

We took full advantage of this break time. I had to relieve myself badly. Conducting a quick surveillance of the area and determining there was no easy way around this, I wondered how I could get some privacy. All of our trucks were packed closely together, and I was the only female on the entire convoy. Our Humvee had a trailer attached to it, and that seemed like the only place I could get somewhat of a cover. I had Candon and Markowitz pull guard for me as I crouched down in between the Humvee and the trailer and relieved myself as discreetly as possible. I then crawled back into the passenger side and started drinking water again. Although it wasn't that hot out at this point, I never really felt hydrated. I was itching to get back on the road knowing in a few hours we would be there.

At about 5:00 p.m., we reached the city limits of Kuwait. As we crossed the border, we could hear the yelling. Soldiers were overwhelmed with excitement. Kids and adults alike on the side of the roads yelled and hollered. They were different here though. They were not yelling for us to go away. They were welcoming us into their country and seemed happy to see us. I got on the radio and asked the convoy commander if we were allowed to give away the dehydrated meals (MREs) that we had not used. They were going to be turned in anyway. He gave me the okay. I then signaled to SPC Candon in the back to toss the MREs out to the kids. It reminded me of Santa Claus at Christmastime. He was tossing the meals out to the left and right sides of the roads. These children were tripping over themselves trying to get the meals. They started to scare me because a few of the kids were running into the road as we were moving to get their hands on some food. I felt bad, but at the same time, it felt so good to give away the small things we take for granted.

The Kuwaiti people seemed different than Iraqis. They even had a different color to their skin. They were darker and seemed better groomed. Their hair looked much thicker and cleaner. The cars that passed us on the road were different now too. They had a lot more American-type cars. The streets were actually full streets with white and yellow lines and two separate lanes.

The air was thinner, and there was a noticeable difference in the exhaust pollution outside. I could feel the difference in the atmosphere. They told us as soon as we got to Camp Victory in Kuwait that we would be allowed to drop our gear and don our desert boonie caps. That was a lot to look forward to. We had had our gear on for three days straight. We were ready to shed some weight.

Arriving at Camp Victory in midevening, the traffic into the camp was horribly backed up, and we sat in it for a couple of hours. I hadn't realized it at the time, but the camp was set up to sustain several thousand soldiers, marines, and airmen, both waiting to deploy to Iraq and those who were redeploying from Iraq and Afghanistan. This was a huge operation.

When we finally got into the gates, it was like a gigantic weight was lifted off our shoulders. We felt the ease of being in a nonhostile place while we were also allowed at this point to drop our gear and put on our soft boonie hats. I was ecstatic. Then it got even better. We pulled up to all these stations that were set up. At each station, there were things you were supposed to get rid of. These items included extra water, fuel, MREs, wood, scrap metal, trash, and most importantly, the ammo station. That was great because we all had seven twenty-round magazines round magazines full of ammo. We could hardly wait to dump it.

We finally arrived at our designated sleep tents. We had a quick orientation of the area. I couldn't believe my ears: "Over there you have the food court, Pizza Hut, Subway, Hardee's, and a Baskin Robbins. We were starving by now.

To the left were the post exchange and the phone and Internet center. It was all right here. I will never forget the faces of all the soldiers when we were released to go eat. Their eyes were wide and smiles were bright. It was a great feeling. We are finally here, and we made it safely. I took a deep breath, fished for my wallet, and tried to decide what I wanted to eat. Realizing I got to *decide* was the best part of all.

THE JOURNEY HOME

WE WERE COMPLETELY spoiled the first two days in Kuwait. All we did was sleep in an overcrowded circus tent, get up to go eat fast food, and come back and read the magazines we had bought at the post exchange.

The time would quickly arrive when there was some hard labor to be done, so we took advantage of the down time we had. I remember so many photos I took of people sleeping in the tent. Not just sleeping, but sleeping in a deep, deep slumber. It was much-deserved sleep.

The third morning in Kuwait, we were woken up about 8 a.m. We were told it was our turn to go take our trucks to the wash rack. They also informed us to take our wet-weather gear and to plan on being soaking wet. I had heard rumors that the civilians inspecting the trucks for cleanliness before they could be loaded onto the ships were real sticklers. My supervisors told us to plan on spending a good five hours on one Humvee.

We all gathered our wet-weather gear and stuffed it wherever we could put it. I had a drinking device called a camel back that had pockets on the outside of it. I packed a protein bar, a pack of cigarettes, and my wet-weather gear. We would only be out there for the night, or so we were told.

We all got back into our original trucks and convoyed about two hours to the wash rack. When we pulled in, we saw a lot of bright lights and tons of trucks being washed by other soldiers. I knew we would probably be waiting for a while.

After we had been parked in line for about three hours, we were told to go to another wash rack about an hour away. By this time, it was almost two in the morning. We convoyed to the other wash rack and sat there for another few hours.

The bus was tiny and there wasn't a lot of room to move around, but everyone eventually fell asleep. In the morning, we were all woken up and moved into a "holding" trailer. We ate MREs for breakfast, and the wait was long and dreadful. We knew we were so close to getting out of there it made the waiting worse. The main task was to get all of our trucks cleaned and turned over to the port civilians. Then we would only have our individual gear to clean before we could load a plane and fly home.

Darkness fell again and we still waited. I saw mostly 4th Infantry Division patches on the soldiers washing their trucks. The entire time we were in Iraq, we fell under the command of the 4th Infantry, so they were in a way our comrades. We could not be too impatient with them because they were doing exactly what we were trying to do—go home.

It was close to one in the morning when we got started. They gave us a safety brief and told us how the operation worked. You clean every crack and crevice of your vehicle, and then you get a guy in a blue hat to do a pre-inspection. After you are cleared on the pre-inspection, you were allowed to have an actual inspector with an orange hat check it out.

The guys doing the safety briefing told us the only open lanes for trucks right now would be for Humvees. We made out because we were in one of the two Humvees in the group. Our vehicle was actually the first one to be put on a lane. I signed out two pairs of goggles, and we put our wet-weather gear on. Sure enough, five minutes later, we were both soaked from head to toe. The water pressure in the hoses was great, and we felt as if we would make good timing.

I was in the back of the truck scrubbing crusted Iraqi dirt out of dents and creases as Markowitz was pressure-spraying the undercarriage. This went on for more than two hours. It seemed as though everywhere I looked there was more dirt. Then it dawned on me why it had been taking people over five hours to get a Humvee turned in. Dirt was flying out from everywhere!

It was seven hours later when we were finally ready for the pre-inspection. I could not believe we had been working on our truck for so long. The time just slipped away. It was now eight in the morning. My skin had turned into raisin bread, and my eyes hurt from sleep deprivation.

I ran around for a while and finally found a blue hat. He checked our truck out and immediately found spaces where there was still dirt. It was like he knew exactly where to look. The places that were so easily overlooked by us he knew so well. All I could do was smile and silently curse at myself. I was frustrated.

It took us three more tries, and finally we passed the pre-inspection. The overall inspection went well. Only minor deficiencies came up, but they were things we could fix on the spot, like scraping some adhesive off the window or a pine needle on the hood. By the time we had our vehicle tagged and moved into the port sterile area, we had been working on it for ten hours straight.

Markowitz and I were exhausted and went inside the bus to sleep. I was in a tiny seat in the back and crunched up between people and gear, but it seemed like the best sleep I had ever had. My feet were still in boots and soaked.

I started to feel my right foot throb, so I took my boots off to air them out.

I awoke to excruciating pain. I looked down at my foot and noticed it had turned a pale-white color and looked waxy. Being a medic, I knew the symptoms of trench foot and was pretty sure that's what I had. I stumbled over to Captain Monti, one of our physician assistants. He confirmed the trench foot, and I thought, *Great, this is all I need right now.*

We waited nearly fourteen hours for everyone else to finish. I had no medication on me, and I was in serious pain. I elevated my foot the best I could and tried to keep it clean and dry. I could barely walk when I had to use the bathroom. I was limping and embarrassed that I would let myself, a medic, become injured.

When we finally collected as a group onto the bus and headed back to Camp Victory, you could see the tears of joy on everyone's faces. We were so glad these three days were over, and the biggest task we were given for redeployment. Now all that waited was our small tasks and getting onto an aircraft to go home.

We returned to the camp and crashed out for the rest of the day. There were still soldiers who came in later than us who still hadn't washed their trucks, but they told us whenever they gather one hundred soldiers who have cleared the wash rack and turned in their vehicles, they will fill a plane. Our group was soon told to pack up to move to the outbound aircraft-holding area. We packed our bags and took the short trip to the out processing center on the camp. It was right on the flight line. We were so close we could hear the planes taking off.

The first station we went to was the briefing for redeploying soldiers. They gave us snacks and drinks, and we listened attentively. They told us things like, "If you have any Iraqi bayonets or ammo, throw them in the amnesty box now." We then went through the customs section. They dumped out our bags and searched through them as they would at an international airport.

Once we were repacked, we had to consolidate all of our bags onto pallets to be loaded on the plane. Shortly, we only had our carry-on bags and our weapons. We were moving quickly with the last-minute details. Now all we had to do was make our way to the refreshment/holding tent and wait for a bird.

Combined with other units from the brigade, there were at least one hundred soldiers in the refreshment tent. I went to the large white cooler, pulled out a Mountain Dew, grabbed my *People* magazine from my carry-on, and sat comfortably in the canvas lounge chair that was provided. I thought, *It can't get much better than this*. I felt a sense of accomplishment. We did everything we were supposed to do, and now it was time to leave. In a way I was sad, but that didn't last long as I was overwhelmed by the idea of lounging this way in my own apartment.

I was in a deep daydream when our platoon sergeant called all the medics to the front of the tent. It was a group-photo opportunity that I could not miss. We all gathered in a small huddle and Kool-Aid grins gleamed on everyone's faces. We were overjoyed and probably had just taken the happiest photo there would be from this deployment. Everyone had their arms around each other. I felt like I was hugging my brothers and sisters. I knew this was, in fact, my second family.

"Okay, listen up! We have a bird on the ground and another en route. You're all getting out of here today."

Those words rang like music to my ears. This was it. It was finally time leave. Tears flowed, blood shed, and sweat poured for this very moment. We felt our courage, strength, and pride overwhelm us all at once. It was an emotional moment that still brings tears to my eyes. Though our mission was still being carried on in Iraq, we had completed our part, and now it was time to say good-bye to Iraq and all that went with it. We were going home.

A HERO'S WELCOME

I HAD NEVER been so relieved to see such bad weather. It was raining and snowing when we stepped off the plane at Aviano Air Base in Italy. It was the first week of March and freezing cold. It didn't seem to bother anyone though.

We all took buses to a large hanger where there was a big bright-yellow banner on the top of the hanger that said "Welcome Home Sky Soldiers." I felt the hero's welcome just from that banner. They say not to get cocky when you return, but I felt in this situation it might take me a bit to adjust to all the attention.

There were wives and families holding flags and banners. They were cheering and hollering as we unloaded the buses. They formed somewhat of a red-carpet entrance into the hanger. The brigade commander was in the line close to the door to shake every soldier's hand as we stepped inside. The applause and cheers were so loud it almost shook me. In a small way, I wished I had my family there to hug me. I felt selfish knowing that was impossible. They were all the way in Florida, and I couldn't even tell them when or where I was going.

We all were in the hanger and seated in rows and rows of chairs facing a highly decorated stage. There were refreshments in the back of the room that some of the wives had put together. There was coffee, soda, and water. I was tired so I grabbed a cup of coffee and sat down.

The brigade commander was the first one to approach the stand. He almost had tears in his eyes as he was praising us for our accomplishments. He gave a speech that was incredibly emotional. He gave thanks to us, the families, and those who gave the ultimate sacrifice in Iraq. When he started naming those who died, I held my breath in negative anticipation. I could hardly keep my tears back. I could only see Craig's face and hear his laugh. I saw Sergeant Yashinski fixing our Internet, and I could see the picture of Specialist Kent's wife in his helmet and his wedding ring on his swollen finger. It took all I had not to burst into tears.

A few others spoke, and most of the soldiers were quiet. I think they were either emotional or just plain tired. I was a little bit of both. I looked around and saw that my fellow medics also appeared sad. I was relieved in a way knowing I wasn't the only one who was so affected by all of this.

Once the briefings and speeches were over, we piled back onto the buses for the two-hour trip to Vicenza, our home base. We made out this time though because we had Italian buses waiting for us. They were luxury buses compared to what we were used to. They had reclining seats, a bathroom, and legroom.

The trip back was exciting. You could feel the tension and excitement. Everyone was cheering and hollering the entire trip. I was looking around and seeing soldiers joking around and really smiling. There were flashes from cameras going off all over the place. One guy sitting in the front even took a picture of the bus driver. I just sat back and smiled. I knew we were getting close.

Once we pulled into the gate, my eyes were being pulled every which way. There were large banners up all over the place for individual companies within the brigade. Most of them were made by the Rear Detachment (those who could not deploy) and the wives of the soldiers who did.

Our banner was the last one on the right side of the gate. It was the best banner I saw out there. It was filled with everyone's nametapes from the company. It read, "Welcome Home 501st FSC." I noticed that all the nametapes were the standard green and the two on the top were desert colored. They read "IVORY" and "YASHINSKI." I clutched my heart and silently thanked them both for their sacrifices.

When we arrived inside the post, I felt several emotions. I was happy, relieved, sad, and guilty. I wanted to be able to say we brought everyone back alive and well, but deep down I knew—this is war, and this is what happens in war. So I took a deep breath and thanked God for returning the remaining paratroopers to our *home away from home.*

THE REALITY
OF HOMECOMING

OUR BUS PULLED up to the welcoming tent. As we all tried to get out of the bus, we had many fans waiting in the streets. Not only were there family members of soldiers, but there were other soldiers from units that did not deploy out there just to shake our hands and welcome us home. I shook a bunch of hands and even hugged a few people I did not know. It felt good. I proceeded to collect my bags and make my way down to our company. They gave us one hour before we were to have formation down at our company dayroom. The married soldiers mingled with their children and spouses, and the singles made their way down the street with their duffel bags and rucksacks.

We were to turn in our weapons, night-vision goggles, and bayonets before formation. I made sure to squeeze in close to the front of the line. I had a lot of things running through my mind now. I felt like I was home but not completely. I wasn't sure where they had parked my car, who had the keys, and if it would even start. Three people had used my car while I was deployed—Billy, his buddy Chris, and then Jose. I found our Rear Detachment NCO, Sergeant Sanders, and asked him where my car was. Luckily, he had my car keys and knew exactly where it was—in the FSC motor pool.

I turned my sensitive items (these are items like weapons and night vision goggles) in and reported to formation. It was brief but to the point. We were dismissed until 0700 hours on Monday for reintegration processing. At one point, I couldn't wait to hear these words; now they echoed in my ear along with car, house, and electric bills. I made my way to my car, which was covered in pine needles by now. I opened the trunk and tossed in my bags. Crossing my fingers, I put the key in the ignition and turned it. Nothing. *Crap.* I knew this was going to be a long night.

I went back to the dayroom and found Sergeant Sanders. He came back to the motor pool and gave me a jump. My car was running now, and I thanked him. Not even five minutes after he left did my car die again; this time I had run out of gas. Whoever was the last person to use my car did not fill up the tank. *Great*, I thought. *That's what I get for being so nice.*

Sgt. Sanders came back again and gave me the keys to his truck and a fuel can. I went to the nearest Agip (Italian gas station) and filled the can with the five euro I had in my wallet. This would be just enough to get home and to another gas station in the morning.

It was over an hour after formation and I was just now heading home. I was afraid of what I would find there. My instincts were right. As soon as I got home, my electric gate opener did not work. There is a key on my key ring that will unlock the gate, so what did I do? I took the keys out and lost my battery charge. It was now 0100 hours and my car was dead, parked in front of my apartment's electric gate. It started to rain and I got back in my car.

Tears streamed my face. I had my Italian phone in my carry-on but the battery was not charged. I had no idea what to do. I knew I couldn't just leave my car blocking the entrance to the gate. I got out and put it in neutral; then I pushed it off to the side as best I could. I jumped the gate and went up to my apartment. I was tired of being in the cold rain.

When I walked in my house, none of the light switches worked, it was freezing, and the apartment carried a nasty mold-type odor. I went downstairs to the main power source and turned my power switch back on.

I made it back upstairs and realized I had left some things in the refrigerator that probably had gone bad. I was never told my power would be shut off, so I figured they must have done this for everyone to conserve the billing.

I pulled out ketchup, a jar of pickles, a pound of hamburger meat in the freezer, and a pack of moldy cheese. Although it was only a few things, I knew the powerful odor would be here for a while. I hadn't even taken off my boots when I began cleaning the inside of my refrigerator. I then went and plugged my phone in and jumped into the shower.

The frustration only grew when I had no hot water. The water became lukewarm for maybe two minutes, and then it was freezing cold. I wanted to scream. I was so frustrated! I kept telling myself, "Tomorrow will be a new day." Covered in goose bumps, I crawled out of my cold shower and into my cold bathrobe. It must have been 40 degrees in my apartment easy. I had no heat, no hot water, and mold growing out of my refrigerator. It was a mess. I was glad to be home but just could not understand why all of this was happening to me. I was angry.

I had to wait until Monday to have my heat turned back on, so I spent the weekend in my sweat pants and layers of shirts and sweatshirts. I slept very little due to the cold and watched TV trying to refrain from the news. It was too hard to watch.

Monday came fast, of course, and we were all back at work at 0700 to start a week on reintegration. This was an interesting program. They had stations set up everywhere, all over post. We had a station for finance, life insurance, promotions, dental exams, medical shots, and anything else that may have been messed up in Iraq or sometime before. There were a lot of lines to wait in. I was very impatient at this point. I just wanted everything to be over with and resume a normal work schedule. People were starting to annoy me.

The first lunch in the food court on post was the first time it really bothered me. I was standing in a very long line for this taco place. There were two soldiers in front of me who couldn't decide what they wanted to order. I was so irritated I almost started yelling, "Just order something, damn it!" I simply kept my mouth shut and bit my lip. They finally ordered after some snickering, and all the while I'm thinking, *These dudes didn't even go anywhere. They sat back here and probably ate tacos every day!* I couldn't believe how angry that made me.

I started talking to my friend Erin about how she felt. The same things were frustrating to her too. It was almost like we were outsiders. The smallest thing would trigger off so much anger and frustration. I felt like those who stayed back didn't understand what we did out there, and I was correct—they never would either.

When a few days went by and we started getting into a system, things started getting a little better. I now had a running car, running hot water, and heat in my place. The post had changed quite a bit. I saw a lot of construction that also irritated me. There was hardly any parking any-where on post. Things just kept adding up to my level of frustration. I was pulling my hair out. Why couldn't they have fixed everything while we were gone? It looked like there were projects they had just started.

Erin and I decided to go to the mall and shop one day after work. We went to two different malls that day. We were ready to spend money, but something funny hap-pened. We walked around for hours and everything looked strange. Clothes were different now—even Italian clothes that we thought were weird to begin with. The only thing I bought was a jacket that had the "Lonsdale" logo printed on it. Lonsdale is a clothing brand name out of London, and I got a kick out of that.

Erin bought nothing. We went to a small bar in the mall and had a beer—the first beer we had had since we had been back. It was good. I had a small buzz off that one beer. We stopped there and hung out for a while talking. The bar was crowded with young Italians. They were talking and laughing and carrying on like no war was taking place. I guess I just figured they didn't care as much because it wasn't their country.

On the way home, I saw a graffiti sign on a cement wall that read "No War, USA." It made me sick. Who are they to say "no war?" Again, I was angry and went home to sleep.

The next few weeks went by very slowly. It seemed as though everything was in slow motion. I couldn't stop thinking about all those soldiers who died and those who came back missing limbs and eyesight. There were so many who gave so much it brought me to tears several nights at a time. I wished I could have done something to save Craig, Ski, and Kent. Those were the three who truly had an impact on my life. The more time I had off, the more time I had to think about it. I was pulling my hair out. I was driving myself crazy.

CLOSURE

IT WAS A month or so after our return that my nightmares started. I was envisioning all those people I cared about whom we lost every day. I wanted to reach up and touch Craig's hand. I wanted to see SGT Yashinski smiling, and I wanted to see Kent hug his wife. These things dwelled in my mind constantly.

The nightmares and lack of sleep lasted for three months. I finally broke down and went to see a counselor. They prescribed a sleeping agent and an antianxiety medication. I was diagnosed with PTSD (post-traumatic stress disorder). This was not an uncommon disorder among soldiers who have been in a combat zone and seen a lot of trauma. I felt embarrassed and ashamed that I could no longer handle what I was feeling.

The first visit to my counselor, I completely broke down. He had no chance to say anything. I just started crying. I hurt for everyone who went and saw what I saw, everyone who went and didn't make it back, everyone who took our place, and the Iraqi children who were brainwashed from their brainwashed parents. I was hurting for the Iraqis who were innocent.

I hurt for my family for worrying about me so much, and I hurt for Billy who worried so much about me. He was always doing whatever he could to make me more comfortable out there. After he left, on our phone conversations he would always say he felt so helpless now. I hurt so badly for him.

Most of all, I just hurt. I grew comfortable and eventually explained everything to my therapist. I told him what I had seen, how it made me feel, and what my reactions were like. He gave me direction and incentive to take my journal from Iraq and write a book. This book was initially written for self-therapy reasons. I finished it a month later. I felt like for once, in the last nine months, I finally had some closure.

18908340R00096

Printed in Great Britain
by Amazon